Breast Cancer
Clear & Simple
All Your Questions Answered

Breast Cancer
Clear & Simple
All Your Questions Answered

From the Experts at the
American Cancer Society

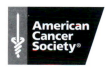

Published by the
American Cancer Society
Health Promotions
250 Williams Street NW
Atlanta, GA 30303-1002

Printed in the United States of America

Designed by Christian Kenesson, Albuquerque, NM
Cover designed by Christian Kenesson, Albuquerque, NM

5 4 3 2   12

Library of Congress Cataloging-in-Publication Data
Breast cancer clear & simple : all your questions answered / from the experts at the American Cancer Society.
        p. cm.
ISBN-13: 978-0-944235-72-0 (pbk. : alk. paper)
ISBN-10: 0-944235-72-7 (pbk. : alk. paper)
1. Breast—Cancer—Popular works. I. American Cancer Society. II. Title: Breast cancer clear and simple.

  RC280.B8B673 2007
  616.99'449—dc22

                        2006018502

For more information about breast cancer, contact your American Cancer Society at **800-ACS-2345** or **www.cancer.org.**

Quantity discounts on bulk purchases of this book are available. Book excerpts can also be created to fit specific needs. For information, please contact the American Cancer Society, Health Promotions Publishing, 250 Williams Street NW, Atlanta, GA 30303-1002, or send an e-mail to **trade.sales@cancer.org.**

Breast Cancer
Clear & Simple
All Your Questions Answered

A Note to the Reader

Reading this book is not the same as getting medical advice from a doctor. This book may not include all possible choices, treatments, medications, safety measures, side effects, or results. For any choices that have to do with your health, talk to a medical doctor who knows your health history. To learn more, call your American Cancer Society at **800-ACS-2345** or go online at **http://www.cancer.org**.

Background and Resources

A Breast Cancer Journey, Second Edition, also published by the American Cancer Society, was a major source for this book. Specific details for information derived from this book and other sources are provided in footnotes throughout the text.

Medical Reviewer
Terri Ades, MS, APRN, AOCN

Plain Language Writer and Editor
Wendy Mettger, MA

Writer
Amy Brittain

Editor
Jill Russell

Managing Editor
Rebecca Teaff, MA

Book Publishing Manager
Candace Magee

Book Publishing Director
Len Boswell

Strategic Director, Content
Chuck Westbrook

Illustrator
Kari Lehr, Birch Design Studios

CONTENTS

*Finding
Out*

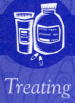

Treating

Recovering

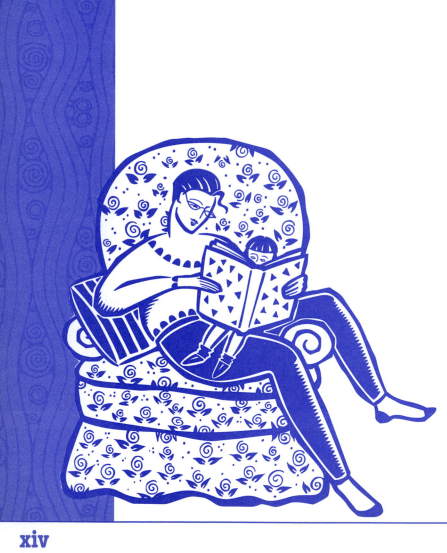

Introduction

About this book

It's important to know what to expect during your breast cancer treatment and recovery. We've written this book to help you

- understand breast cancer;
- learn how it may affect you;
- find out about your treatment choices;
- face problems with money, work, or your home life;
- recover from breast cancer; and
- get your life back.

We answer many common questions about breast cancer. We also suggest some questions you may want to ask your doctor. We encourage you to ask these questions and discuss your choices with your doctor.

How to use this book

This book is divided into two sections.
The first section takes you step-by-step through

- **finding out** you have breast cancer—
  the diagnosis *(die-ug-NO-sis)*;

- **treating** your breast cancer; and

- **recovering** from treatment.

The second section—"More Information"—gives
you more information about cancer diagnosis and
treatment, as well as helpful resources.

There is a lot of information in this book. Read
only what you want to right now. Use the
"Contents" section at the front of the book to
help you quickly find what interests you. The
"Resources" section on pages 156–165 tells you
where to find more information and support.
Also, a glossary on pages 166–169 has definitions
of medical terms.

Finding Out You Have Breast Cancer

The doctor told me I have breast cancer. What do I do now?

You may be in shock. You may feel angry, worried, overwhelmed, hopeless, or scared. In fact, you may not know what to do. That's okay. It's normal to be upset and confused. No one wants to hear that she has breast cancer.

Don't rush.

You may feel like your cancer must be treated right now, even if you aren't sure how. But learning more about your breast cancer first can help.

Reading this book might be helpful to you. Take a few days or weeks to talk to your doctor and learn about your treatment choices. That way, you can make sure you're making the best decisions for you and your health.

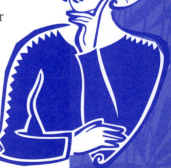

What will happen to me?

Will I be okay?

Each person's cancer is different.

Most women with breast cancer are treated and live. In fact, two million women in the United States have had breast cancer and are alive today.

You may already know family members and friends who have had breast cancer, were treated, and went on with their lives. These women are proof that there is life after breast cancer treatment for most people.

Experts are working on better ways to find and treat breast cancer all the time.

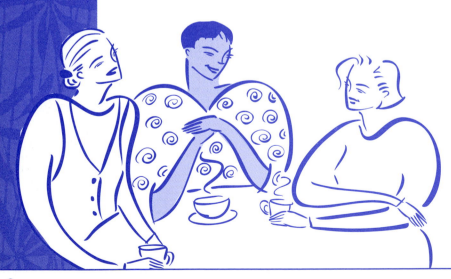

Will I lose my breast?

Most women do not lose a breast.

Doctors can often remove the breast cancer without removing the whole breast. They take out the cancerous lump and some of the breast tissue around the cancer. This is called a lumpectomy *(lump-EK-tuh-me)*.

What if I do need my breast removed?

Some women do need their whole breast removed to get all the cancer.

Removing one breast is called a mastectomy *(mas-TEK-tuh-me)*. Removing both breasts is called a double mastectomy.

It is very upsetting to lose one or both of your breasts. You will need support and information to help you cope with your loss. Read more about mastectomy and coping after a mastectomy on pages 42–43.

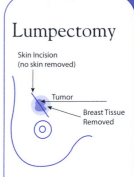

Lumpectomy

Skin Incision
(no skin removed)

Tumor

Breast Tissue
Removed

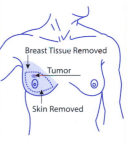

Total Mastectomy

Breast Tissue Removed

Tumor

Skin Removed

Source: Surgical treatments for breast cancer. From Exploring treatment options. *A Breast Cancer Journey*, 2nd ed. Atlanta, GA: American Cancer Society; 2004:102.

Will I be in pain?

Having cancer does not mean you have to be in pain.

If you do have pain from cancer or cancer treatment, there are many ways you can feel better. You do not have to suffer through any pain you feel. Medicines and some ways of relaxing can help. Here are some suggestions:

- **Talk to your doctors about any pain you feel.** The more doctors know about your pain, the better job they can do to relieve it. Don't be afraid to talk about your pain.

- **Ask for help with your pain.** Getting relief from your pain can help you deal with your cancer. Being free of pain will help you stay strong so you can get through your cancer treatment.

- **Don't feel you have to choose between getting treated for cancer and getting treated for pain.** Doctors can take away your pain while also treating your cancer.

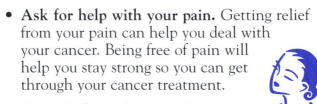

My friend had breast cancer. Will the same things happen to me?

Each woman with breast cancer is different.

What happens to one woman with breast cancer will not happen to all women with breast cancer. Here are a few reasons why:

- **Breast cancer affects people in different ways.** Not everyone with one type of cancer has the same experience.

- **There are different kinds of breast cancer.** They affect the body in varied ways.

Doctors don't treat every breast cancer the same way. They think about your breast cancer and your health. Then they make a special treatment plan for your cancer. Your doctors will make a treatment plan just for you.

My loved one had another kind of cancer.

Should I expect the same things to happen to me?

Not all cancers are the same.

You've probably known someone who has had cancer. Just because something happened to that person does not mean it will happen to you. There are several reasons for this:

- Some types of cancer, like breast cancer, can be treated more easily than other types.

- Some types of cancer and cancer treatments make people sicker than others.

- Some types of cancer are found when they are small and easier to treat. Others are found later, after they have been growing for a while, and are harder to treat.

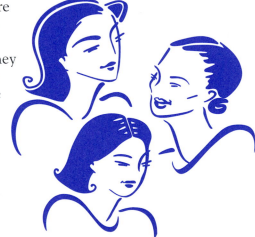

- People often have other illnesses that affect how they respond to the cancer treatment.

What is breast cancer?

All living things, from plants to people, are made up of tiny cells. The healthy cells in your body grow, form new cells, and die when they're supposed to.

But cancer cells are not normal and do not follow the patterns they should. They don't die like other cells. They keep growing, making new cells, and spreading in the body. In breast cancer, these cells grow out of control and form a lump called a tumor (*TOO-mer*).

Here are more facts about breast cancer:

- When doctors find breast cancer before it grows into a large tumor or spreads, they can treat it more easily.

- There are different types of breast cancer. Not every breast cancer grows the same way, and doctors don't treat every breast cancer the same way.

- Breast cancer mostly grows in women, but men also can get breast cancer.

> For information about different types of breast cancer, call the American Cancer Society—Toll-free: **(800)ACS-2345.**

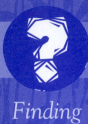

Why me?

Am I to blame for my breast cancer?

No. It's not your fault you have breast cancer.[1]

Many women want to know why they got breast cancer. Some women think they caused their cancer. They may think they got breast cancer as a punishment for something they did or didn't do. Or they may think if they had done something differently, they wouldn't have breast cancer. You did not cause your breast cancer.

We don't know what makes most breast cancer start to grow. We do know that some things in a woman's life affect her chances of getting breast cancer. This is called her "breast cancer risk." But even if they increase a woman's chances of getting breast cancer, no one has proved that they cause breast cancer.

For more information about breast cancer risk, see pages 139–144.

[1] See Endnotes, page 170.

If I don't feel sick, do I really have cancer?

Cancer doesn't always make you feel sick.

Some women say they can't believe they have cancer because they feel fine. It can be hard to accept that you have breast cancer when you don't feel any different. Other women may not feel quite right for a while before doctors find their breast cancer.

Cancer can grow for a long time before it spreads and causes problems or pain. That's why getting checked regularly for cancer is so important. The earlier cancer is found and treated, the better a person's chances for a long life after treatment.

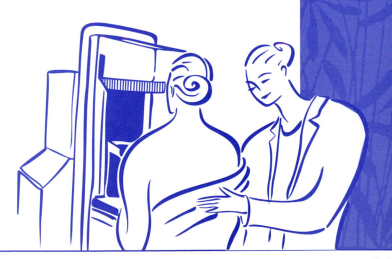

How serious is my cancer?

How do doctors know how serious my cancer is?

They study the lump in your breast.

Doctors study your breast tissue sample (taken out during your biopsy) and write a pathology (*path-AWL-uh-gee*) report. It explains the type of breast cancer you have and how big the tumor is. It also states whether your tumor is likely to grow quickly or slowly.

Doctors use the report as a guide to help them plan how to treat your cancer. The pathology report uses a system of numbers and letters to show how serious your cancer is and to decide your "cancer stage." For more information about cancer staging, see pages 146–149.

The doctor says my breast cancer has spread. What does that mean?

It's possible for cancer to move to another part of the body.

Sometimes cancer cells break away from a tumor and spread to other parts of the body. They can settle in other places in the body and form new tumors. This spreading is called metastasis *(meh-TAS-tuh-sis)*.

Even when cancer has spread to a new place in the body, it is still named after the part of the body where it started. If breast cancer spreads to the lungs, for example, it is still called breast cancer. Breast cancer is most likely to spread to the lungs, bones, liver, or brain.[2]

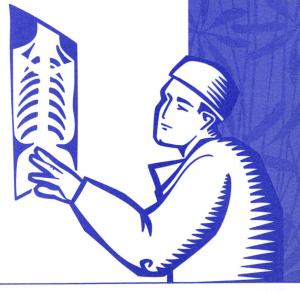

What does "cancer grade" mean?

"Cancer grade" shows how likely it is that your cancer will grow and spread quickly.

When doctors talk about "cancer grade," it is one way of talking about how serious your cancer is.

To figure out the grade of your cancer, doctors look at your cancer cells under a microscope. They give your cancer a grade from 1 to 3. Cancer grades are described as

- **grade 1**, or low grade;
- **grade 2**, or intermediate grade; and
- **grade 3**, or high grade.

Grade 1 cancer cells look the most like healthy, normal cells. They are less likely to grow and spread quickly. Cancer cells that are grade 3 look the most different from normal cells. They are more serious and could grow more quickly.

What does "cancer stage" mean?

"Cancer stage" means how much cancer is present and if it has spread.

Doctors use the term "cancer stage" to describe

- the extent of your cancer;
- if your cancer has grown; and
- if your cancer has spread to other parts of your body.

Doctors use a system of letters and numbers to describe how much your cancer has spread. They use this information to decide your cancer stage. The cancer stage helps your doctor make treatment plans and also figure out what is likely to happen with your cancer.

See pages 146–149 for more information about cancer staging.

How big is the tumor?

The drawings below will give you an idea of how big the lump in your breast is. They show breast tumors that range in size from one centimeter to five centimeters.

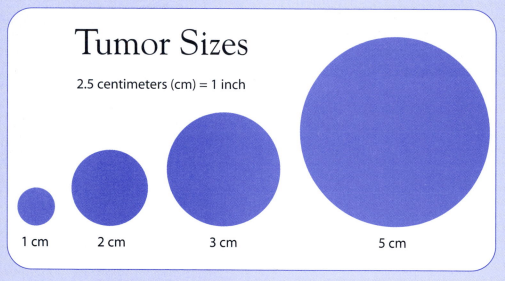

Tumor Sizes

2.5 centimeters (cm) = 1 inch

1 cm   2 cm   3 cm   5 cm

Source: *Breast Cancer Treatment Guidelines for Patients*, Version IV/September 2002. Courtesy of the National Comprehensive Cancer Network (NCCN) and the American Cancer Society (ACS).

Does my doctor know how well I will respond to treatment?

Your doctor may be able to predict how you will respond to treatment.

Your doctors study what has happened to other women who had the same cancer stage and grade you have. They find the latest information on how many women with breast cancer like yours have had the same treatment. Then they see how well treatment worked for these women. With this information, they can help predict how you might do with treatment.

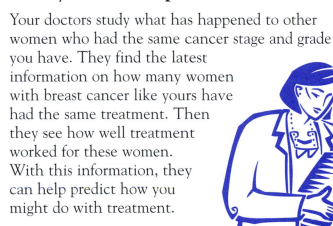

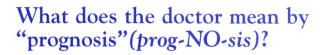

What does the doctor mean by "prognosis" *(prog-NO-sis)*?

The doctor is talking about what will probably happen with your cancer.

Prognosis is a prediction of how well you will do during the course of your cancer treatment and afterwards. It relates to your chances of recovering from cancer and living after cancer treatment.

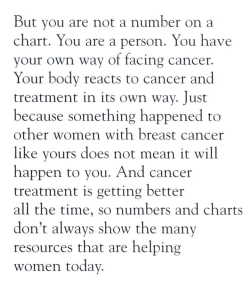

But you are not a number on a chart. You are a person. You have your own way of facing cancer. Your body reacts to cancer and treatment in its own way. Just because something happened to other women with breast cancer like yours does not mean it will happen to you. And cancer treatment is getting better all the time, so numbers and charts don't always show the many resources that are helping women today.

Why doesn't the doctor use the word "cure"?

Because it's hard to know if every cancer cell is gone forever.

Most doctors use the word "remission" instead of "cure." They will say, "Your cancer is in remission." This means that tests done after you have completed cancer treatment don't show any cancer. It is a wonderful moment for many women.

However, a few cancer cells might still be hidden somewhere in the body and start growing later. That's why doctors don't like to use the word "cure." They cannot guarantee that the cancer is completely gone.

Many women recover completely from breast cancer and have no sign of any cancer being present. Other women are able to keep their cancer under control and live long lives.

Do I need a second opinion?

Consider getting a second opinion. It can be helpful to hear what another doctor says about your breast cancer.[3]

You may want to talk to another doctor about your diagnosis and the treatment plan your first doctor suggested. This is called getting a second opinion.

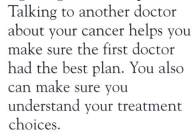

Talking to another doctor about your cancer helps you make sure the first doctor had the best plan. You also can make sure you understand your treatment choices.

How do I get a second opinion?

Start by getting recommendations from others.

You may want to ask the doctor who gave you the cancer diagnosis for names of other doctors you could see. You also can ask for help getting in to see these other doctors. Some women choose to get a third opinion.

After talking with different doctors, think about what you have learned. Talk it over with friends and family members. Then choose the best treatment for you. Once you make that decision, it's time to start your breast cancer treatment.

If you have health insurance, it may pay for you to see a doctor for a second opinion. Talk to your insurance company before you go to another doctor.

Won't the first doctor be mad if I want to talk to someone else?

Doctors understand why you want a second opinion.

Wanting a second opinion doesn't mean you think the first doctor gave you poor treatment or advice, or that you don't trust the doctor. It means you want to know more and get the best treatment.

Many doctors will encourage you to talk to another doctor about your biopsy, your cancer, and what is likely to happen. They know that your health and life are at stake. They also know you should feel as comfortable as you can with the diagnosis and treatment plan.

If your doctor gets mad or refuses to suggest another doctor, then you need to think about whether he or she is the right doctor for you.

Questions to ask the doctor who told you about your cancer

1. What is the grade of my breast cancer?

2. What could this cancer grade mean for my health and my life?

3. What is the stage of my breast cancer?

4. How does my cancer stage affect which cancer treatments I should have?

More questions on next page

5. How does my cancer stage affect my prognosis?

6. Could you explain the different parts of my pathology report to me?

7. I'd like a second opinion. How do I get one?

8. Can you recommend a doctor to give me a second opinion?

9. How do I get my biopsy samples to that doctor?

10. What other tests do you think I will need?

Treating Your Breast Cancer

Who will help with my cancer treatment?

Can I choose my doctor?

You may be able to choose who will be in charge of your cancer treatment.

Talk to your doctor about finding an oncologist (*on-CALL-uh-jist*). This is a doctor who treats people with cancer. You will want to find an oncologist who has treated a lot of women with breast cancer.

Most hospitals have more than one doctor who treats breast cancer. These doctors may be experts in cancer, surgery, or radiation treatment. Your oncologist will most likely oversee all your treatment.

What should I think about when choosing a doctor?

Think about what you want most from a doctor.

You will be with your cancer doctor (oncologist) for quite some time. He or she will give you your treatment. And you will continue to see your oncologist for regular checkups years after treatment. It is really important to find a doctor you trust.

Here are some questions that may help you choose your doctor:

- Does the doctor explain things in a way you can understand?
- Does the doctor listen to your concerns and questions?
- Does the doctor treat you with respect?
- Do you and the doctor share a common approach to your health and breast cancer treatment?
- Can you reach the doctor when you need to ask questions or get other information?
- Has the doctor treated a lot of women with breast cancer like yours?

Most doctors only work at certain hospitals. Your decision about which doctor to see may be closely tied to the hospital where he or she works. See the next question for more information on hospitals.

Where will I go for treatment?

It's most likely that you will get treatment at the hospital or clinic where your oncologist works.

Most doctors only work at certain hospitals. A good doctor usually works at a good hospital. Find out if the hospital where your doctor works treats a lot of women with breast cancer. Ask if the hospital is well known for its good treatment of women with breast cancer.

You can ask your oncologist and family doctor these questions. They will help you feel comfortable about the hospital where you will get care.

Who else will care for me?

There will be many people caring for you during your cancer treatment.[4]

You will see doctors, nurses, and other medical staff trained to help women with breast cancer. This flow chart shows the people who may be part of your treatment team. See pages 150–154 for descriptions of the medical team members.

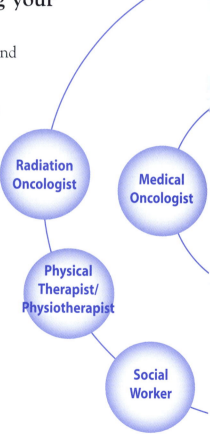

Radiation Oncologist

Medical Oncologist

Physical Therapist/ Physiotherapist

Social Worker

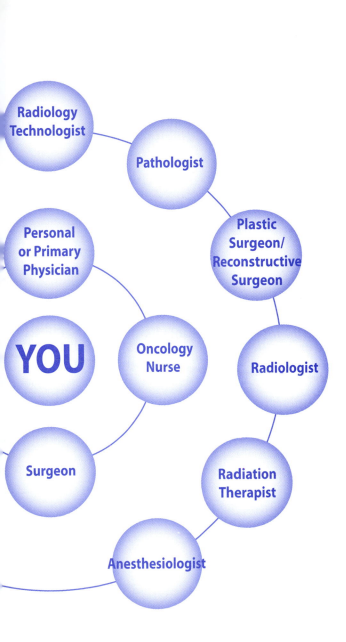

Source: Medical Team Flow Chart. From Making the medical system work for you. *A Breast Cancer Journey, 2nd ed.* Atlanta, GA: American Cancer Society; 2004:67.

Questions to ask a doctor who may treat you

1. What is the exact type of breast cancer I have?[5]

2. Have you treated this type of breast cancer before? If yes, how many times?

3. When is your office open?

4. Who would take care of me if you were on vacation or if I needed help when the office was closed?

5. Can I bring someone with me to take notes?

6. Where would I be treated (which hospital)?

7. Does this hospital treat a lot of women with breast cancer?

8. Do they use the best, most current breast cancer treatments?

9. Are you willing to talk to my family members about their concerns?

10. Do you have information about breast cancer I can take with me?

11. Where can I find more information about breast cancer?

How to talk to your doctor

It is not always easy to talk with your doctor. You may feel worried, think your questions are silly, or just feel too tired to talk. Also, your doctor may be in a rush. You may get the feeling that he or she doesn't have time or want to answer your questions. All these issues can make it hard to talk to your doctor.

Here are some tips to help you feel more comfortable talking to your doctor and asking questions:

- Make a list of questions to ask your doctor.
- Understand that there are no "stupid" or "silly" questions.
- Let the doctor know right away that you have questions.
- Take notes of what your doctor says.
- Have someone come with you to help ask questions and take notes.

Why ask questions?

Your doctor knows a lot about cancer. Talk to him or her and find out about your breast cancer treatment. Questions are important for these reasons:

- You need to understand what is going on.
- You should know why the doctor thinks you should have a certain treatment.
- You want to make sure you agree with the treatment suggestions.

Asking questions doesn't make you a bad patient. It is your doctor's job to help you get better and to explain what is going on.

Make sure you understand

The words doctors and nurses use to talk about cancer can be hard to understand. They may use words you have never heard before. Here are some tips to help you understand what they are saying:

- Ask them to explain the word.
- Ask them to draw a picture to explain the word or concept.
- Ask them to give you an example from everyday life to help explain the word.

Work as a team

The more you can talk to your doctor and get answers to your questions, the better you can work together as a team during your breast cancer treatment. Working as a team will help you get good care.

What's the best way to treat my breast cancer?

What kind of treatment will I get?

There are many ways to treat breast cancer.

Your doctor will suggest a special treatment plan for you. Your plan may include one or more of the following treatments:

- Surgery
- Radiation therapy
- Chemotherapy
- Hormone therapy
- Monoclonal antibody therapy

How do I know if doctors are suggesting the best treatment?

Talk to your doctor about what treatments have worked best for your type of breast cancer.

Ask why he or she is suggesting certain kinds of treatment. Are these treatments the most effective for your type of breast cancer? Ask for more information (breast cancer education materials, articles, and good Internet resources) about the treatment your doctor suggests. This information can help you make decisions about your breast cancer treatment.

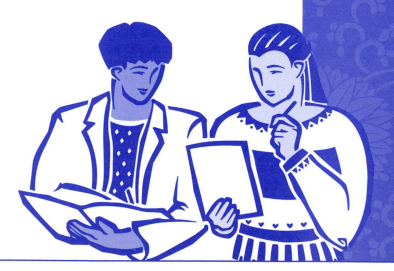

How is surgery used to treat breast cancer?

Doctors do surgery to cut the cancer away from healthy breast tissue.

Surgery is one of the most common treatments for breast cancer. During surgery, the doctor may remove the cancer with a small amount of breast tissue, or she may need to remove one or both of your breasts. These two kinds of breast cancer surgery are called lumpectomy and mastectomy.

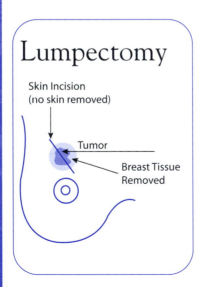

Lumpectomy

Skin Incision
(no skin removed)

Tumor

Breast Tissue
Removed

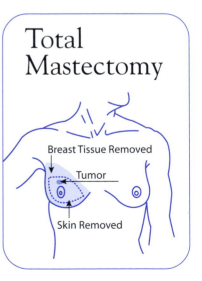

Total Mastectomy

Breast Tissue Removed

Tumor

Skin Removed

Source: Surgical treatments for breast cancer. From Exploring treatment options. *A Breast Cancer Journey*, 2nd ed. Atlanta, GA: American Cancer Society; 2004:102.

- **Lumpectomy** is removing the lump, or tumor, and some of the breast tissue around it to treat the cancer. If cancer is found at the edge of the tissue (removed by lumpectomy), the surgeon may need to remove more tissue. It is important to have a clear, cancer-free margin of normal breast tissue to avoid recurrence.

- **Mastectomy** is removing the full breast or both breasts in order to treat the breast cancer.

Sometimes during surgery for breast cancer, lymph (*limf*) nodes are taken out as well. Lymph nodes are small bean-shaped areas of tissue that help fight infections in the body. Cancer can spread through the lymph nodes. The doctor checks your lymph nodes to see if the cancer has spread.

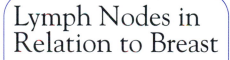

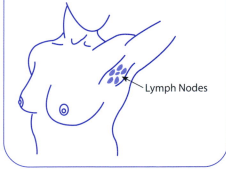

Source: Lymph nodes in relation to the breast. From What is breast cancer? *A Breast Cancer Journey, 2nd ed.* Atlanta, GA: American Cancer Society; 2004:15.

How do I decide between the two types of surgery?

Think about how each type of surgery will affect your life.

Talk to your doctor about your choices.

Here are some questions to help you decide which surgery is best for you:

- Which surgery does your doctor suggest and why?

- How would you feel about losing one or both of your breasts?

- What if you need radiation therapy after your lumpectomy? What's involved in radiation therapy? (See page 46 to read more about radiation therapy.)

- What if you decide to have breast reconstruction surgery after your mastectomy to rebuild your breast? What's involved? (See page 109 to read about options after a mastectomy.)

See pages 39–41 for more questions to ask your doctor about surgery.

More questions to ask the doctor about surgery

1. What are the risks and benefits of each type of surgery?

2. Would one surgery or the other lower the chances that my cancer would come back?

3. What side effects should I expect from each surgery?

4. How would my breast look after a lumpectomy?

5. How would my breast look after a mastectomy?

6. Do you have photos you can show me?

7. What are my choices for making it look like I have two breasts if I have a mastectomy but don't want more surgery?

What should I expect after a mastectomy?

A mastectomy usually takes two to three hours.[6] After the surgery, you will probably stay in the hospital for one or two nights. Doctors and nurses will check to make sure you are healing well.

When you wake up after surgery, you will see a bandage over your breast area. You also may have one or more tubes called drains in your breast or underarm area. These stay in place for about a week. The drains remove fluids that collect while you're healing.

You will need to see your doctor a week or two after surgery.

Women are often surprised by how little pain they have in the breast area after surgery. But you may have strange feelings like numbness, pinching, or pulling in your underarm area.

Talk with your doctor about how to take care of yourself after surgery. Before leaving the hospital, you should get a printed form telling you what to do. If not, ask about the following:

How to take care of your body:

- How to take care of the wound and bandage
- How to take care of the drains
- How to know if you have an infection
- What medicines to take (including pain medicines) and how often
- When to call your doctor or nurse

How to get back into your life:

- What to eat and what not to eat
- What activities you should or should not do
- How soon you can return to work

How to get used to your body after surgery:

- When to start using your arm
- How to exercise your arm to keep it from getting stiff
- When you can wear a breast form (padding shaped like a breast that can be worn under the clothing)
- What to do about feelings you may have about how you look
- How to get in touch with an American Cancer Society Reach to Recovery® volunteer. Reach to Recovery is a program in which breast cancer patients can talk by phone or face-to-face with breast cancer survivors.

What should I expect after a lumpectomy?

A lumpectomy, also called breast conserving surgery, takes less than one hour.[7] Most of the time, you have a lumpectomy as an outpatient and do not have to stay overnight in the hospital.

After a lumpectomy, you may have a drain put in your armpit. This is usually taken out before you leave the hospital. Sometimes the drain needs to stay in longer and may be removed at your follow-up visit with your doctor (about one week after surgery).

You will need radiation treatment after your lumpectomy. You receive radiation treatment for up to seven weeks after surgery, usually five days per week. If you are getting chemotherapy, your doctor may want you to wait to get radiation therapy.

Women are often surprised by how little pain they have in the breast area after surgery. But they may feel numbness, pinching, or pulling in the underarm area.

Most doctors want you to start moving your arm soon after surgery so it won't get stiff.

Talk with your doctor about how to take care of yourself after surgery. Before leaving the hospital, you should receive a printed form telling you what to do. If not, ask about the following:

How to take care of your body:

- How to take care of the wound and bandage
- How to take care of the drains
- How to know if you have an infection
- What medicines to take (including pain medicines) and how often
- When to call your doctor or nurse

How to get back into your life:

- What to eat and what not to eat
- What activities you should or should not do
- How soon you can return to work

How to get used to your body after surgery:

- When to start using your arm
- How to exercise your arm to keep it from getting stiff
- How to get in touch with an American Cancer Society Reach to Recovery volunteer. Reach to Recovery is a program in which breast cancer patients can talk by phone or face-to-face with breast cancer survivors.

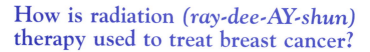

How is radiation *(ray-dee-AY-shun)* therapy used to treat breast cancer?

Radiation therapy uses special x-rays to kill or harm cancer cells.

There are two main ways radiation therapy may be used to treat breast cancer:

- A special machine is used to point powerful x-rays at the cancer from outside the body.

- Tiny pellets containing the radiation are put into the body where the cancer is. The radioactive pellets are placed directly into the breast tissue next to the cancer.

Radiation hurts cancer cells, but it also hurts healthy cells. This can cause side effects such as muscle stiffness, mild swelling and tenderness, and a sunburn-like reaction on the skin where you received radiation. These side effects should go away as the normal, healthy cells recover. See pages 56–57 for more about side effects.

Radiation therapy may be used before surgery to shrink a tumor. It is also used after surgery or chemotherapy to destroy any cancer cells that could be left behind. A woman usually has treatment five days a week for up to seven weeks. Each treatment lasts a few minutes and doesn't cause pain.

How is chemotherapy (kee-moh-THAYR-uh-pee) used to treat breast cancer?

Chemotherapy uses drugs to kill or harm cancer cells.

There are two main ways chemotherapy is given:

- By having a needle placed in your arm. The liquid chemotherapy goes through the needle and attacks cancer cells in your body.

- By taking pills that contain the chemotherapy medicine.

Chemotherapy drugs stop cancer cells from growing and dividing. Like radiation therapy, chemotherapy can also affect healthy cells. This can cause some side effects. Common side effects include nausea, vomiting, feeling tired (called fatigue), and low blood counts. These side effects should go away as the normal, healthy cells recover. See pages 56–57 for more about side effects.

Chemotherapy may be used after surgery to kill any cancer cells still in your body. A woman having chemotherapy for breast cancer usually takes two or more different chemotherapy drugs for three to six months.

How is hormone therapy used to treat breast cancer?

Hormone therapy uses drugs to change the way hormones work in the body. It helps stop cancer cells from growing.

Hormones are chemicals made in the body. Certain kinds of breast cancer need hormones so they can grow. If the hormones are blocked, cancer cells can't grow.

Hormone therapy is used after surgery to lower the chances of cancer coming back. It also is used to treat breast cancer that has spread to other parts of your body. Sometimes it is used with chemotherapy.

Based on the tests done on your breast cancer tissue, your doctor will know if you have the type of breast cancer that will be likely to respond to this treatment.

How is monoclonal antibody (*ma-nuh-KLO-nul ANN-tih-bah-dee*) therapy used to treat breast cancer?

Monoclonal antibody therapy helps the body fight cancer cells.

Some kinds of breast cancer need certain proteins to grow. Monoclonal antibodies keep these proteins from working right. If the proteins don't work right, the cancer cells can't grow.

Monoclonal antibodies are like proteins, but are made in a lab and then put into your body. Unlike chemotherapy or radiation therapy, monoclonal antibodies can be used to find and hurt only cancer cells. They don't hurt healthy cells.

They may be used as the only treatment or with chemotherapy. From the tests done on your breast cancer tissue, your doctor will know whether you have the type of breast cancer that will be likely to respond to this treatment.

What should I know about herbs, dietary supplements, or special diets used to treat cancer?

These treatments don't cure cancer.

When you have cancer, you may want to believe that there is a magic way to fix it. But when something sounds too good to be true, it usually is. There isn't an herb, supplement, or diet that will cure cancer. If you are thinking about adding an herb, supplement, or special diet to your cancer treatment, please talk to your doctor first. Find out about how the vitamins, herbs, or other therapies might affect your cancer treatment and if they cause side effects.

Your doctor needs to know about any supplement or medicine you take. It's a safety issue.

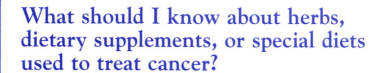

Help making your treatment choices

Your doctor has probably given you a lot of information about treatment. You may feel overwhelmed by your treatment choices. In fact, some women prefer to have their doctors make their treatment decisions. Other women want to learn all they can and then make their own choice. Whatever you decide is okay.

If you want to be involved in your treatment decisions, here are some questions to ask:

- **The facts**—how effective is this treatment for your breast cancer?

- **Treatment**—what will happen to you during treatment and how will it affect your life?

- **Side effects**—what are the possible side effects from this treatment?

- **Other women with breast cancer**—is there someone you could talk to who has been through the same treatment?

No one expects you to become an expert on cancer treatment. But you may feel more in control if you understand your choices and what may happen.

The American Cancer Society's Reach to Recovery volunteers can talk to you over the phone or in person about cancer treatments and also share their own experiences with you. Call **800-ACS-2345 (800-227-2345)** for more information.

What is a clinical trial?

It is a type of research study.

Clinical trials test medicines and/or procedures to see if they are safe and can help people.

Thousands of people take part in clinical trials each year. Your doctor may want you to think about being part of a clinical trial. Ask your doctor why she thinks it might help you and what you can expect to happen during the study.

A person must be matched with a clinical trial. For example, to be part of a breast cancer clinical trial, a woman will need to meet these requirements:

- Have a certain stage and grade of cancer
- Be within a certain age range
- Not yet have received treatment
- Have already received a certain treatment

There are benefits and risks to being in a clinical trial. Here are some good things that may happen if you take part in a clinical trial:

- You may get great care that other people cannot yet get.
- You may get lots of attention from doctors who want to give the best care possible.

- You may help other people by letting doctors learn more about how to treat your type of breast cancer.

Here are some bad things that may happen if you take part in a clinical trial:

- You do not get to choose the treatment you get.

- Your health insurance may not cover the cost of the care you get.

- You may need to travel to the clinic a lot and get many tests.

- Your treatment may cause side effects that doctors don't yet know about.

Remember: taking part in a clinical trial is your choice. No one can force you to take part. You also can drop out of a clinical trial if you decide it's not right for you.

For more information about clinical trials, call the American Cancer Society at **800-ACS-2345 (800-227-2345)**. You also can visit our Web site at **http://www.cancer.org** and search for "clinical trials matching service."

Questions to ask the doctor about treatments

1. Which treatment(s) do you think would work best for my cancer?

2. Will the treatment(s) help me live longer?

3. Will the treatment(s) make my life better? If so, how?

4. How well does the treatment(s) usually work on my type and stage of breast cancer?

5. Are there other treatments we can try if this one doesn't get rid of my cancer? If so, which ones?

6. When would the treatment(s) happen and for how long?

7. Would I need to stay in the hospital for treatment? If so, for how long?

8. What steps would I need to take to get ready for treatment?

9. What are the possible risks or problems of this treatment?

10. How will you know if the treatment is working?

11. When do I need to make my treatment decision?

What do I need to know about side effects from treatment?

What are side effects?

Side effects are unwanted symptoms or problems that happen because of treatment.

Most cancer treatments cause side effects. Here's why. These treatments are strong enough to kill your cancer cells, but they also harm the healthy cells in your body. As your healthy cells are harmed, you may feel sick, tired, or lose your hair. Most of these side effects go away after your treatment is over.

There are ways to help prevent or stop some side effects. Ask your doctor about these issues:

- The possible side effects of the treatment he or she is suggesting for your cancer

- How likely it is you will have side effects

- What can be done to prevent the side effects or deal with them if you get them

- How long the side effects will last

- If the side effects will go away after your treatment is done

Doctors often talk about common side effects and less common or rare side effects caused by chemotherapy. Here's a list of both:

Common Side Effects

- feeling sick to your stomach
- not feeling hungry
- a change in the foods you like
- hair loss
- feeling tired
- dry or sore mouth
- easy bruising or bleeding
- a greater chance of infections

Rare Side Effects

- damage to your heart, liver, and kidneys
- hearing loss
- nerve damage in your hands, feet, and legs
- having a second cancer later in life

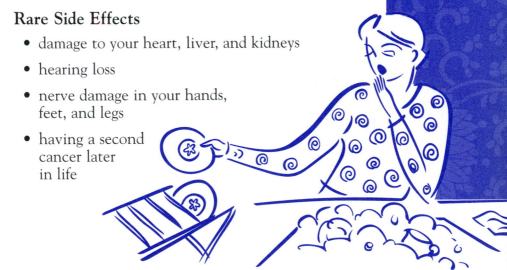

Will treatment make me feel sick?

Cancer treatment can make you feel sick to your stomach. It also can change your taste or desire for food.

What happens:

A few minutes or hours after you have chemotherapy, you might throw up or feel sick to your stomach. Sometimes radiation therapy and 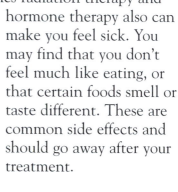 hormone therapy also can make you feel sick. You may find that you don't feel much like eating, or that certain foods smell or taste different. These are common side effects and should go away after your treatment.

What you can do:

Ask your doctor about medicines you can take to help you feel better. You also may want to try the tips below.

What to eat:

- Eat foods without much taste, like dry toast and crackers.

- Try popsicles or Jell-O.

- Slowly sip cold, clear drinks like ginger ale.

- Eat foods with smells you like, such as lemon drops or mints.

How to eat:

- Eat small meals all day.

- Eat food cold or at room temperature. It has less smell and taste than hot food.

- Try to rest for an hour after you eat a meal.

- Try to relax and take slow, deep breaths when you feel sick.

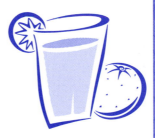

Will I lose my hair?

Some cancer treatments may make you lose your hair, but it grows back.

What happens:

Many women lose their hair after a few weeks of chemotherapy, and some lose it during hormone therapy. Other women have problems with thinning hair, but don't lose all their hair. Some women lose hair from their eyebrows, eyelashes, and hair from other parts of their body. How much hair you lose depends on which chemotherapy drugs or hormone therapies you take, how much of them you take, and how long you take them.

Many women worry about losing their hair because of cancer treatments. This is normal. Not many of us are comfortable with hair loss. Our hair has a lot to do with how we feel about ourselves.

If you lose your hair, it will almost always start to grow back after your treatment. Sometimes when hair grows back, it is a different color or has more curls than it had before.

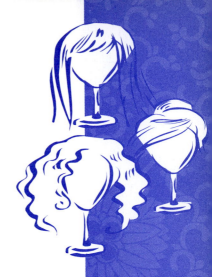

What you can do:

Here are some ideas to help you cope with hair loss:

- Think about cutting your hair short before it starts to fall out.

- Call your health insurance company to find out if they will pay for a wig. Then ask your doctor for a prescription for a wig.

- Choose a wig before treatment starts or early in your treatment if you want to match your hair color and texture.

- Ask your doctor or nurse for a list of wig shops, or look in the phone book. The American Cancer Society's "tlc" catalog has lots of hats and wigs. Call **800-ACS-2345 (800-227-2345)** to request a catalog.

- Wear a pretty hat, turban, or scarf instead of a wig.

- Wear sunscreen to protect your bare scalp, and wear a hat in cold weather to keep in body heat.

Will I feel tired?

Some people in cancer treatment feel really tired.

What happens:

Cancer treatments can make you feel very tired. This feeling, called fatigue (*fuh-TEEG*), is the most common side effect of cancer treatment. Fatigue is different from the feeling you get when you haven't had enough sleep. It is more like your brain, body, and emotions are all tired.

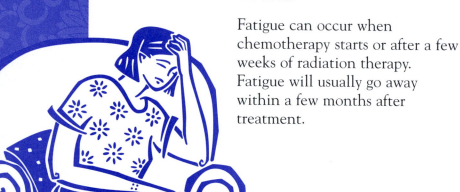

Fatigue can occur when chemotherapy starts or after a few weeks of radiation therapy. Fatigue will usually go away within a few months after treatment.

What you can do:

If you feel really tired, try the steps below:

- Take care of yourself.
- Get enough sleep.
- Eat well.
- Ask your doctor about drugs that might help.
- Exercise if you can—it may give you more energy.

Set limits:

- Don't make yourself do more than you feel you can.
- Decide which things are most important for you to do. Get lots of rest and save your energy for those things.
- Let other people help you.

What is lymphedema (limf-uh-DEE-muh), and will I get it?

Lymphedema is swelling of the arm. It can start after some treatments that affect the lymph nodes in your underarm.

What happens:

Lymphedema is a buildup of fluid that causes the arm to swell. The amount of swelling varies for each woman. Some women may have swelling that makes their rings feel tight on their fingers. For other women, it can make their arm swell to twice its normal size.

Lymphedema may start right after surgery or radiation therapy, or may happen months to years later. Most often, it sets in slowly over time. It occurs in women who have had lymph nodes removed during surgery or who have had radiation therapy to the lymph node area. About one out of every five women who have had breast cancer will get lymphedema.

How to lower your chances of getting lymphedema[8]:

- **Try to avoid infection.** Have blood drawn and shots given on the arm not affected by surgery. Keep the skin clean and protect it when you have cuts, scratches, or burns. Wear gardening gloves when gardening.

- **Try to avoid burns.** Protect your arm from sunburn. Use oven mitts when cooking. Avoid splash burns from microwaved and steaming foods. Don't use hot tubs and saunas. The heat can cause fluid buildup.

- **Try to avoid clothing or other items that squeeze or put pressure on the affected arm or shoulder.** Avoid using shoulder straps when carrying briefcases and purses. Have your blood pressure taken on the other arm (or on the thigh when both arms are affected). When traveling by air, wear a compression sleeve (a custom-made bandage worn on the arm to reduce swelling) to protect against changes in pressure. Talk to your doctor or physical therapist about whether you should be fitted for a sleeve.

- **Try to avoid muscle strain.** It's okay to do your normal activities with the affected arm, but don't overdo it. Exercise, but try not to overtire your arm. Talk with your doctor about the level of activity that is right for you.

What you can do:

If you have had lymph node surgery or radiation therapy to lymph nodes in the underarm area, watch for signs of lymphedema. Look at your upper body in front of a mirror every two weeks. Call your doctor if you notice any of these signs:

- A full or tight feeling in your arm

- The arm on the side of the body where your cancer was treated looks bigger than the other

- Weakness in your arm or not being able to move it as far as before

- Skin changes, like skin that stays pushed in after you press on it

Call the American Cancer Society at **800-ACS-2345 (800-227-2345)** for more information about how to take care of your arm and lower your chances of getting lymphedema.

Could I have other side effects?

Yes. Ask your doctor about other possible side effects.

After chemotherapy, you might have a hard time thinking or remembering things. You may hear this called "chemo brain." Or you may have sores in your mouth. Ask your doctor what you can do about these side effects. These are other possible side effects:

- **Skin and breast changes.** Radiation therapy can make your skin red like a sunburn, make your skin feel thicker, or change the size of your breast. These changes usually go away six to twelve months after treatment. Chemotherapy can make your skin red, itchy, dry, or peel.

- **Hair loss from any part of the body and not just the head.** Hair loss from chemotherapy occurs over a period of days to weeks. After chemotherapy, the hair grows back.

- **Getting sick more easily.** Some treatments can weaken your body so that you get sick, bleed, or bruise more easily than before.

- **Hot flashes, vaginal discharge, and other effects of hormone therapy.** Other side effects may include vaginal dryness and/or itching, irregular menstrual periods, headache, nausea, skin rash, fatigue, and weight gain.

- **Changes in how you go to the bathroom.** You might be constipated or have diarrhea during chemotherapy.

- **More chance of getting another cancer.** It is very rare, but sometimes treatment can make another cancer grow in your body. If this should happen, it would be years after your breast cancer treatment.

Is there help for any pain I might have?

Yes. Doctors can help you feel better if you are in pain.

Tell your doctor about any pain you feel. Pain can be a sign that something is wrong in your body. Let the doctor know when the pain started, how long it lasts, and if anything makes it better or worse. Also, tell the doctor how bad your pain is on a scale of one to ten, with one as the lowest amount of pain and ten as the very worst pain. And follow these steps:

- **Take your pain medicine when the doctor tells you to.** Do not wait until the pain is really bad to take your medicine. It is easier to stop pain before it starts or keep pain under control than to get rid of serious pain once it starts.

- **Tell your doctor about any side effects you have.** Pain medicines may make you feel sick or constipated, but other medicines or laxatives can help with these problems.

- **Do not stop taking your pain medicine all at once.** Ask your doctor before stopping. He may have you take a little less each day until you are off the medicine.

There are many pain medicines. If one pain medicine doesn't work for you, talk to your doctor about trying another. You should get enough pain relief to be able to do the things that are important to you.

Can I cope with side effects like pain without medicine?

There are many ways you can feel better without medicine.

The methods below may help you deal with side effects or just feel better. You can get information on these and other ways of helping your mind and body from your doctor, by calling the American Cancer Society, or from books, videos, and Web sites. You also may be able to find classes at gyms and community centers. Some hospitals and health centers can train you in these techniques or help you find professionals who do them.

- **Acupuncture** (*AK-you-punk-chur*) can help with nausea from chemotherapy. A professional inserts very thin needles into specific places in the skin.

- **Aromatherapy** (*uh-roam-uh-THER-uh-pee*) can help with pain, depression, and stress. Essential oils (fragrant substances from plants) are either inhaled or massaged into the body.

- **Hypnosis** (*hip-NO-sis*) can help lower blood pressure and help with pain, fear, anxiety, nausea, and vomiting. It is a way of putting people in a state of relaxed alertness that helps them focus on a certain problem or side effect.

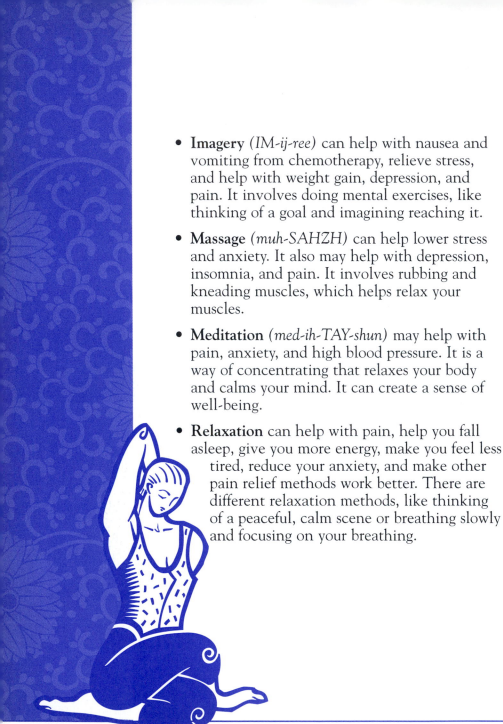

- **Imagery** *(IM-ij-ree)* can help with nausea and vomiting from chemotherapy, relieve stress, and help with weight gain, depression, and pain. It involves doing mental exercises, like thinking of a goal and imagining reaching it.

- **Massage** *(muh-SAHZH)* can help lower stress and anxiety. It also may help with depression, insomnia, and pain. It involves rubbing and kneading muscles, which helps relax your muscles.

- **Meditation** *(med-ih-TAY-shun)* may help with pain, anxiety, and high blood pressure. It is a way of concentrating that relaxes your body and calms your mind. It can create a sense of well-being.

- **Relaxation** can help with pain, help you fall asleep, give you more energy, make you feel less tired, reduce your anxiety, and make other pain relief methods work better. There are different relaxation methods, like thinking of a peaceful, calm scene or breathing slowly and focusing on your breathing.

- **Spirituality** can help by lowering your stress and anxiety and helping you have a more positive outlook. It is an awareness of something greater than a single person and usually involves religion and prayer.

- **Tai chi** (*tie chee*) can lower your stress, heart rate, and blood pressure levels. Tai chi is an exercise that involves movement, meditation, and breathing. It may help with posture, balance, building muscles, flexibility, and strength.

- **Yoga** can help relieve some symptoms of cancer. Yoga is a type of exercise that involves different postures and breathing. It can help you relax and get physically fit.

Remember, there is no one "right" way to treat your pain. It's okay to try medicine and some of the methods listed above for pain relief. You need to find out what works for you.

Will I be able to have children after treatment?

It depends on the type of cancer treatment you get.

Ask your doctor **before** treatment if you will be able to have children after treatment. Some chemotherapy drugs can make you unable to have children for a while or forever. Any problems you have getting pregnant after treatment will depend on these factors:

- How old you are during treatment

- How much chemotherapy you have and for how long

- Which chemotherapy drugs you take

Ask if there is anything you can do before treatment that could help your chances of having children after treatment.

Questions to ask the doctor about side effects

1. What are the possible side effects of this treatment?

2. How long might side effects last?

3. Will I feel tired or sick during treatment?

4. Will any of the side effects change how I look, either for a short time or for good?

5. Could another treatment fight my cancer but affect my life in a different way?

More questions on next page

6. Which side effects should I expect right away?

7. Which side effects should I expect later?

8. What side effects should I call you about right away?

9. Can anything be done to stop side effects before they start or lessen them?

10. How should I take care of my skin, breast, or body during treatment?

11. Are there any services or programs that can help me cope with side effects?

How can I pay for treatment?

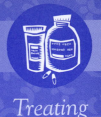

What if I don't have health insurance?

You may still be able to get help paying for your health care.[9]

Medicare and Medicaid, government health insurance programs, may help with some of your costs (see page 77). We've also listed other government programs that may help pay for your health care. See the "Resources" section on pages 156–165 to find out how you can contact these groups and get more information.

- **Medical assistance programs:** These programs may help people who make less than a certain amount of money pay for health care. Ask your hospital social worker or case manager about programs in your state.

- **Drug assistance programs:** The groups NeedyMeds and the Pharmaceutical Research and Manufacturers Association of America (PhRMA) can give you information about programs that help pay for medications.

- **Hill-Burton Program:** Some hospitals and medical centers offer free or low-cost care to people who can't pay. Each center decides what medical care it will offer for free or lower cost.

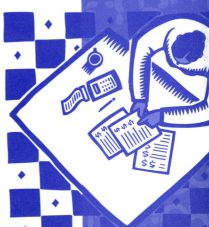

- **National Breast and Cervical Cancer Early Detection Program:** Some states offer free testing for breast cancer through the National Breast and Cervical Cancer Early Detection Program (NBCCEDP). If you were checked for breast cancer through this program and have cancer, NBCCEDP may pay for your treatment.

- **Veterans' benefits:** If you are a veteran of the armed forces or married to a veteran, you may be able to get health care through the Department of Veterans Affairs.

Ask your hospital social worker about these programs. Check with your local county hospital and find out which services it offers for people who don't have health insurance. The American Cancer Society also can talk to you about your insurance or financial needs and help you find resources.

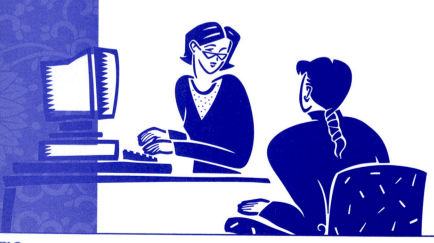

What do Medicare and Medicaid pay for?

These government programs pay for some of your medical care, but not all of it.

You must first qualify for Medicare or Medicaid before they will pay for any of your medical care. You may be able to get Medicare if you are sixty-five years or older or if you get Social Security benefits because you are disabled. You may be able to get Medicaid if you make less than a certain amount of money or are disabled.

It can be confusing to figure out what medical costs are covered by these programs. Call Medicare at **800-633-4227** or visit their Web site at **http://www.medicare.gov** to find out which cancer treatment and medicines are covered. You also can ask a social worker or case manager at your hospital or call the American Cancer Society at **800-ACS-2345 (800-227-2345)** with questions.

Are there private groups that can help me pay for my treatment and other costs?

There are private groups that may help you pay your treatment and other living costs.

Talk to the social worker at your hospital. Or call the American Cancer Society at **800-ACS-2345 (800-227-2345)** for information on how to get help from these organizations:

- **Community groups** such as the Salvation Army, Catholic Social Services, United Way, Jewish Social Services, and others

- **National groups** like Eldercare Locator, which helps senior citizens, and CancerCare, which offers help and information about paying for expenses and other practical help

The "Resources" section at the back of this book has more information about groups that may help.

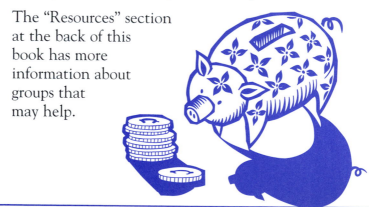

What if I can't pay my bills?

Explain what is happening. Ask for more time or other help.[10]

Many people have a hard time paying bills at one time or another. It is nothing to be ashamed of. Most hospitals and other companies will listen to your story and try to help. Try taking the steps below:

- Ask to pay the bill later or in a few payments instead of one.

- Explain the problem to hospital billing staff. Ask about payment options.

- Talk with a social worker at the hospital about ways you can get help for a while with money challenges.

- Think about letting relatives or friends help out with money for a little while. If they know what you're going through, they may want to help. It may be hard to accept this type of help. But by helping you, your friends and family may feel they are helping with your recovery from cancer.

What is private health insurance and what does it pay for?

Private health insurance is insurance you get through work or that you pay for on your own. These plans may pay for many treatment costs.

The medical care, drugs, and supplies that health insurance pays for are called "benefits." If you have health insurance, look at the terms of your policy and make notes about what is and is not paid for. Insurance may not pay for prescription drugs, counseling, or care in your home. Ask if you can get more insurance benefits through a catastrophic illness clause.

What if my insurance claim is turned down?

Ask for help. The insurance company may still cover your claim.

The bills you or your doctor sends to the insurance company for payment are called claims. Keep track of your bills and send claims to your health insurance company as soon as you get them. Hospitals, clinics, and doctors' offices usually have someone who can help you fill out claim forms.

Sometimes an insurance company will not pay one of your medical bills. If this happens, ask your doctor's office or the hospital claims office for help. They may be able to look at the claim form and find the problem. Also, call your insurance company and find out how to "appeal" a claim that has been turned down. This means that you submit the claim again and ask the company to pay.

Keep copies of important papers: claims, "letters of medical necessity," bills, receipts, requests for sick leave from work, and any letters to and from the insurance company. These records will help you get payment for your medical bills.

Questions to ask the hospital billing department

1. How much will my cancer treatment cost?

2. Will I get separate bills from the hospital, surgeon, and other doctors?

3. Is this treatment covered by most insurance plans?

4. How much of the costs will my insurance cover?

5. If I don't have insurance or the treatment isn't covered
    by my insurance, are there any ways I can get help
    paying for it?

What is a breast cancer "survivor"?

Many women choose to think of themselves as breast cancer survivors. "Survivor" is a word some people use to mean anyone who has been diagnosed with cancer. Someone living with breast cancer could therefore be called a "breast cancer survivor." Other people use the word "survivor" to mean someone who has finished cancer treatment or who has lived several years after a diagnosis of cancer.

Not everyone thinks of herself as a survivor. Some people would rather not be called a "survivor." This is a personal choice.

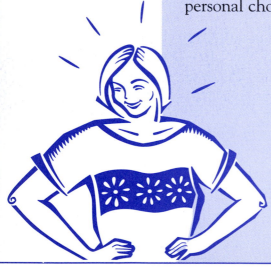

How will cancer and treatment affect me and my loved ones?

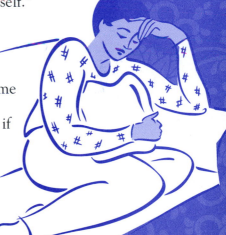

Does anyone feel the way I do?

Yes. Many women feel confused and upset about having breast cancer.[11]

It's normal to be worried, sad, or angry.

Here's how some women with breast cancer feel:

- "I feel like I will be a burden to my family if I take time to go to doctors, if I'm not feeling well, or if we have to pay for treatment."

- "I worry about my family and how upset they will be more than I worry about myself."

- "I worry about how to talk to my children about my breast cancer."

- "I worry that my partner will leave me or that future partners won't think I'm pretty because I have cancer or if I've had a breast removed."

- "I'm afraid of what will happen in my life and what will happen to my body."

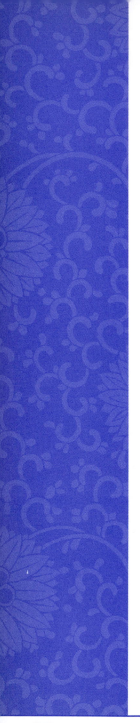

You might have some of these same worries. Don't be too tough on yourself. It is hard to adjust to having cancer and getting treatment. It affects so many parts of your life. You are bound to worry sometimes. You will feel happier on some days than others.

If you feel really down and find yourself thinking about death or killing yourself, you may have what is called clinical depression. This is very serious. Tell your doctor right away if you have any thoughts or feelings like this.

How can I feel more in control of my life?

Think about ways you can deal with your fears or challenges.

It might help to think through what worries you, then think of ways you can deal with each of your fears or challenges. For example, if you're worried about how you would look without your breast, talk with women who have had mastectomies. Ask them about their experiences. Find out what they did to cope with their mastectomy. Your concern might have to do with seemingly "less important" everyday tasks. Maybe you're worried that vacuuming will hurt your arm and that you won't be able to do it. You could ask a friend to help you with chores, or you could trade less active chores with a friend or neighbor.

Any worry you have is perfectly okay—every woman is different, and no concern is silly.

Think of the things that worry you—whatever they are—and write them down. Then write down as many ideas as you can that may help you feel more in control. Think about who can help you.

Start with your biggest worries:

1. I'm afraid or worried that _____

   _____

   What are all the ways I can think of to make this

   better? _____

   _____

2. I'm afraid or worried that _____

   _____

   What are all the ways I can think of to make this

   better? _____

   _____

3. I'm afraid or worried that _____

   _____

   What are all the ways I can think

   of to make this better? _____

   _____

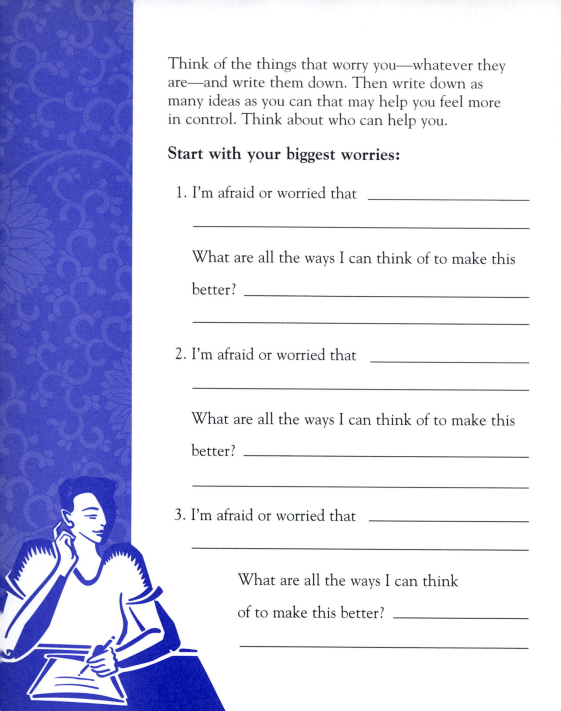

Keeping a journal may help

Think about keeping a journal. It's a helpful way to get out feelings like anger, confusion, fear, or guilt.

Write down what happens in your life. Describe what it feels like to have cancer. Write about how other people react to the news that you have cancer. Write about what happens when you see the doctor or how you feel about your treatment choices.

Writing about your feelings may help you cope with your cancer and feel better. You may want to begin writing in your journal by finishing the sentences here.

1. When I first found out I had cancer, I felt _____

   _____

2. I wish that I _____

   _____

3. I can make this happen by doing _____

   _____

4. One of the things I worry about most is _____

   _____

Continued on next page

5. What would make me feel better is _____

_____

6. When I tell other people about my cancer _____

_____

7. I feel closest to other people when _____

_____

8. I get upset when _____

_____

9. When I get mad I _____

_____

10. When things get to be too much I _____

_____

11. I would like to deal with things by _____

_____

12. I couldn't get through this without _____

_____

13. The best times I have are _____

_____

14. What I like most about myself is _____

_____

How can I find help and support?

There are many places that can help you.

Going to support groups with other women who have breast cancer can be a way for you to

- talk about your feelings, your fears, and the changes in your life;

- hear what has happened to other women and learn from them;

- spend time with women who understand what you're going through; and

- learn about other kinds of help in your area.

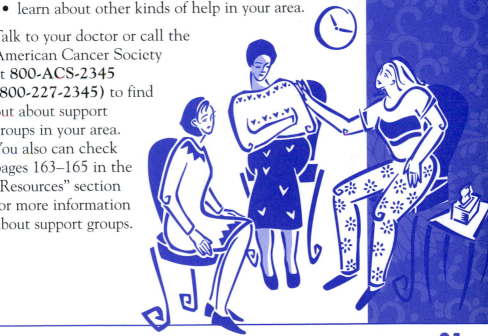

Talk to your doctor or call the American Cancer Society at **800-ACS-2345 (800-227-2345)** to find out about support groups in your area. You also can check pages 163–165 in the "Resources" section for more information about support groups.

I told my family that I have breast cancer. Why are they acting strangely?

Family members may act strangely because they are afraid.

Family members may not know how to act. Their fears probably are related to

- worries about losing you;

- what will happen to them if something happens to you;

- not knowing how to help you;

- worrying about not being strong enough when you need them; and

- worries about the cancer itself.

You may be able to help them by talking about what you think will happen, how you feel, and how treatment may affect you. If you want, let them know they can ask you questions and talk to you about your cancer. This may help all of you feel more comfortable. If you need help talking with your children about your cancer, please call the American Cancer Society at **800-ACS-2345 (800-227-2345).**

How will cancer affect my friendships?

Friends will react to your news in different ways.

Some friends will offer help right away or try to make you feel better. Others may stay away from you because they don't know what to say or do. They may be afraid of what may happen to you. Or they may worry that they might say the wrong thing. Some may even think they can catch cancer from you. (This can't happen. People don't get cancer from another person.) Some friends may be upset if you don't feel well enough to spend time with them or go to get-togethers.

It is natural for friends to want things to be like they used to be, before you had cancer. Read the next section to find out how to talk with your friends about your cancer.

How can I talk to family and friends about cancer?

Try to be honest and let them know what's happening.

If it feels okay, let friends and family members know these facts:

- That you have breast cancer (they may feel hurt if they hear the news from someone else)

- That you expect to go through treatment and live

- That you can't give them cancer

Let them ask questions and tell them what you've learned about breast cancer. If someone says something that hurts your feelings, let that person know. But try to understand if people seem to act funny or distant. Like you, they're figuring out what to say and how they feel.

If you aren't comfortable talking about personal things, it's okay not to open up about your feelings or your cancer.

How will cancer treatment affect my life at home?

You may not be able to do everything you used to do.

Your daily life may need to change because of your cancer treatment. You may feel tired or sick and just not have much energy. This means that you'll need to do less at home and others will need to do more. Talk with your family members and friends about how they can help.

Give them something specific to do. Ask them to pick up the kids from school, do the dishes, bring over a meal, or run to the drugstore. Let them know that you'd like to talk about things other than cancer for a while. Or ask them just to sit and relax with you. People can help more when they know what really makes you feel better.

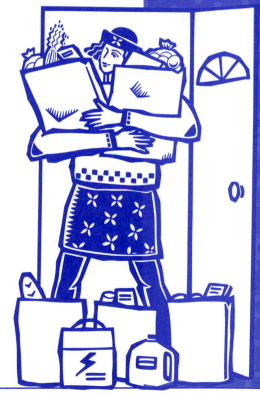

Can anyone help me with day-to-day challenges?

Special programs and trained staff may be able to help.

There are programs that can give you rides to the doctor, help you find child care, or even pay bills and solve insurance problems. Talk to your doctors, nurses, or social workers about the type of help you need. Find out who can help.

Some hospitals have staff who are trained to help you find what you need. They may be able to help you

- get to and from your treatment;
- find child care; and
- find other resources in your community that can help.

The American Cancer Society can tell you about local help. Our staff are trained to listen to you, learn your needs, and put together a plan of action just for you. Call the American Cancer Society at **800-ACS-2345 (800-227-2345)** for more information.

Questions to ask the doctor about life during treatment

1. How will treatment affect my day-to-day life?

2. Will I need someone to drive me to and from treatment?

3. What changes should I expect at home during treatment? For example, will I need help with chores, have to cut back on my hobbies, or make other changes to my daily life?

4. How should I take care of my breast, skin, or surgery scar?

More questions on next page

5. What else should I know about taking care of myself during treatment?

6. Will I have energy during treatment?

7. Will I be able to exercise?

8. Will I be able to leave town during treatment?

How will cancer and treatment affect my work?

Is it better to work during treatment or take time off?

If you have a choice and feel well enough, you may choose to continue working.[12,13]

Talk with your doctor about how your cancer treatment might affect your work. Ask if you should take time off from your job.

Many women want to feel as normal as possible during treatment. They choose to go back to work as soon as they can. Some women who have a lumpectomy for early-stage breast cancer do not have side effects that stop them from going back to work. They sometimes work during radiation treatment or go back to work a few days after surgery. Other women take time off to let their bodies and minds rest. Not everyone feels ready to work during treatment or so soon after surgery. Only you and your doctor can decide what you are ready for.

Remember, there is no right or wrong decision about choosing to work or not to work during your treatment. Whatever you decide is okay.

Should I tell people at work that I have cancer?

You may want to if you will be taking time off.

It's up to you to decide how much to tell your coworkers about your breast cancer. They may be helpful and understanding, or they may feel uneasy and not know what to say or do.

If you think telling people at work will be a problem, first talk with a social worker at the hospital. He or she may be able to help you decide how much information you should share.

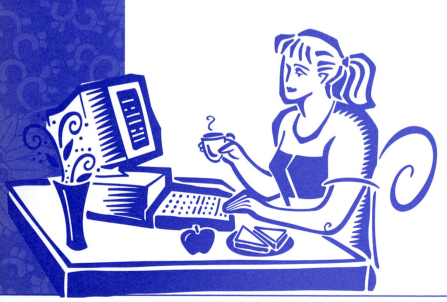

Could I lose my job if I have to take time off?

If you need to take time off, there are ways to protect your job.

You may not even want to tell your employer that you have cancer. But if you need to take time off for treatments, think about telling your employer why you will be gone. Talk with your boss about how much time you expect to take off.

It's a good idea to keep track of all talks you have with your boss or with people in the benefits office. If you think you have been treated unfairly at work, call the Equal Employment Opportunity Commission (800-669-4000).

There are Federal laws that may protect your rights and your job while you are in treatment:

- **The Americans with Disabilities Act (ADA)** makes it against the law for an employer to punish you for having a disability like cancer. The ADA may also protect you if you are looking for a new job. To learn more, call **800-514-0301** or visit the ADA Web site at **http://www.ada.gov**.

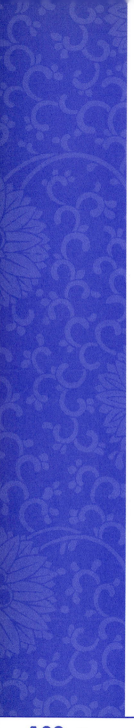

- **The Family and Medical Leave Act (FMLA)** says that employers with fifty or more workers have to give workers up to three months of unpaid time off to take care of themselves or a family member. To qualify, you must have worked at least one year and 1,250 hours. For more information, call the Wage and Hour Division of the U.S. Department of Labor at **866-4USWAGE (866-487-9243)** or visit their Web site at **http://www.dol.gov/esa/whd/**.

How can I get ready to take time off from work?

A little planning will help you and your coworkers.

Before you take time off, discuss these options with your boss:

- Working different hours, working part time, or calling in

- Sharing work with other people

- Passing work on to others

- Making detailed lists of your projects and what needs to be done

- Letting people know the status of your projects

Any of these options may make it easier for you to take time off from work.

Can I get help with money if I'm not able to work?

You may have options for help.

Social workers or case managers at your hospital or organizations like the American Cancer Society can usually tell you about government programs that could help. Patient advocates or financial aid counselors at the hospital may also provide options.

You may not think of yourself as disabled, but the programs below also help people being treated for cancer:

- **Long-term disability insurance:** If you can't work, find out if you have a long-term disability insurance policy through your job. This may give you sixty to seventy percent of your pay.

- **Social Security Disability Income (SSDI):** If you have been working for many years, SSDI may help you. Contact the Social Security Administration (**800-772-1213** or **http://www.ssa.gov**) to find out how to apply. If you get turned down the first time, you can reapply. Any benefits will not begin until you have been disabled six months.

- **Supplemental Security Income (SSI):** If you have not worked much or if you haven't earned very much, SSI may help you. You must be disabled, over sixty-five years old, and/or blind. Ask the social worker at the hospital or your local Social Security Administration office how to apply.

Questions to ask the doctor about work

1. Will I need to take time off from work?

2. If I need to stay home after treatment, how long will I be away from my job?

3. If I do go back to work, will I need a different work schedule?

More questions on next page

4. Will I have a hard time doing any part of my job after treatment?

5. How will I know if I am overdoing it at my job?

6. Do I need to give my employer special forms before taking time off from work?

Recovering from Treatment

What if my breast was removed?

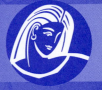

Will I ever get used to the changes in my body?

It takes time, but most women do adjust to these changes.

Cancer and treatment can change the way you feel about your body and yourself. This is normal. You have been through a serious illness and your body is different. After a while most women do get used to their new bodies. They realize that women are beautiful and feminine whether they have two breasts, one breast, or none. But this takes time. Most women are able to accept these changes within one or two years of treatment. For some women it takes longer. Each woman is different.

Give yourself time, and try the following steps:

- **Be patient.** If you can't touch your scars or look at them right away, don't worry. You may need to try many times to feel okay with the change.

- **Play up a part of your body that you like.** You may like to wear skirts or tights to draw attention to your legs.

- **Try to feel good about your whole body.** Just because one part of your body has changed does not mean you are ugly or less of a woman.

- **Don't be hard on yourself.** You don't have to feel happy about the changes. Don't fake it.

- **Join a support group.** Ask your doctor or a social worker at the hospital about support groups for women who have had mastectomies. Talking to other women who have been through the same thing can be really helpful and comforting.

What are my choices after a mastectomy?

You have some choices after a mastectomy:

- **Doing nothing** to recreate your breasts

- **Wearing a prosthesis** (*pross-THEE-sis*) or "breast form," which is shaped like a breast or part of a breast. It can be worn in your bra to fill it out after breast surgery.

- **Breast reconstruction,** which is surgery that can rebuild the shape of a woman's breast, including her nipple and areola (*uh-REE-uh-luh*), the dark area around the nipple.

Some women are okay with having one breast or no breasts and do nothing. Other women feel better using breast forms to fill out their bras and make it look like they have two breasts when they wear clothes. Still other women have breast reconstruction as soon as they can. The choice is yours.

How can I look like I have two full breasts if I don't want surgery to make a new breast?

One option is wearing a breast form.

A breast form or prosthesis is usually heavy enough to match the weight of your remaining breast. It keeps your bra in place, helps your clothes fit better, and balances the weight of your other breast so you don't have backaches. Breast forms give you a natural look. Some can even be worn while you're swimming or exercising. They may be made of silicone, latex, or foam.

If you have had a double mastectomy, you can choose breast forms that will maintain a similar breast size.

If you have had a lumpectomy or are small-breasted, you may want only a breast enhancer. They come in different sizes and shapes and are usually weighted a little bit. You can put one in your bra to make the breast on which you had surgery match the size of your other breast. Putting a shoulder pad in your bra may also work, although it works best if you sew the pad into your bra.

What should I know about a breast form?

You need to know how to find and pay for a breast form.

- **Find out about costs.** Breast forms can be expensive. If you have health insurance, it should pay for a breast form or prosthesis and bra. Medicare and Medicaid also may pay for some of these expenses.[14] If so, find out where Medicare or Medicaid says you need to buy the breast forms. Make sure the bills for your breast forms or bras are marked "surgical" before sending in claims.

- **Ask your doctor to write a prescription** for your breast form and any special bras. This can help you get payment from insurance.

- **Find out if you need a special bra.** Not every woman needs a special bra with a pocket to hold a breast form in place. Sometimes pockets can be added to bras you already have. Many stores sell pocket materials or precut pockets. Some will even sew pockets into your bras for you.

- **Make an appointment with a trained fitter** at the store before you go.

- **Try on different types** of breast forms while you're wearing a comfortable support bra. The most expensive breast form may not be the best fit for you.

- **Be sure the breast form matches your remaining breast** as closely as possible from the top, bottom, and front.

The American Cancer Society's "tlc" catalog sells breast forms and other products for women with cancer. To request a catalog or for more information on breast forms, call **800-ACS-2345 (800-227-2345)**.

What is breast reconstruction surgery?

It is surgery to rebuild your breast.

Here's a list of possible breast reconstruction choices. Talk to your doctor about which might work for you.

- **Breast implants:** The doctor puts padding under your skin where the breast tissue was removed. This fills out the shape of your breast. This is the most common type of breast reconstruction. Implants may be filled with saline (salt water) or silicone gel. People used to worry about whether silicone implants were safe, but studies have shown that both types of implants are safe.

- **Flap procedures:** A doctor uses tissue from somewhere else in your body to make what looks like a breast. The tissue can come from your stomach, back, hip, or buttocks.

Following are diagrams of two types of flap procedures.

The *LAT flap* procedure uses muscle and skin from your back. The muscle and skin are moved to your chest and shaped into a breast.

The TRAM flap procedure uses extra tissue and muscle from the lower abdominal wall. The skin, fat, blood vessels, and muscle tissue are moved from the abdomen to the chest area. The flap is then shaped into the form of a breast.

Continued on next page

- **Nipple reconstruction:** Tissue for the nipple and areola is often taken from your body, usually from the upper inner thigh, and shaped into a nipple. Or small flaps of skin on the reconstructed breast can be brought together to form the nipple. Once the skin heals, a cosmetic procedure involving tattooing may be done to match the nipple of the other breast and to create the areola.

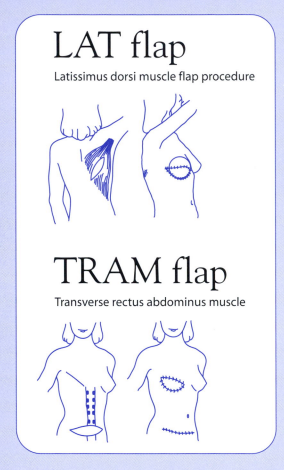

LAT flap
Latissimus dorsi muscle flap procedure

TRAM flap
Transverse rectus abdominus muscle

Source: Flap procedures. From Breast reconstruction. *A Breast Cancer Journey, 2nd ed.* Atlanta, GA: American Cancer Society; 2004:168–169.

Can I have breast reconstruction surgery?

Most women can have surgery to rebuild the shape of their breasts.

You should be able to have this surgery whether you are young or older. If you think you want to have breast reconstruction surgery, discuss this with your doctor before you have your surgery for your breast cancer. Talking about it early will give you more choices for your breast reconstruction.

After you have talked with a plastic surgeon about breast reconstruction, you may want to get a second opinion from another surgeon. You will want to choose which option will work best for you and your lifestyle.

What should I know about breast reconstruction?

Talk to your doctor about what to expect and the side effects you might have.

Ask your doctor questions about breast reconstruction. You also can talk to an American Cancer Society Reach to Recovery volunteer who has had breast reconstruction (**800-ACS-2345** or **800-227-2345**). Keep in mind the facts below:

Breast reconstruction is expensive. The Women's Health and Cancer Rights Act says that health plans that pay for mastectomies also have to pay for breast reconstruction. In addition, health plans must pay for prostheses. To find out more about your rights, call the U.S. Department of Labor with questions (**866-444-3272**) or go online to **http://www.dol.gov/ebsa/publications/whcra.html**. Or call your State Insurance Commissioner's office (look in your phone book in the state government section).

Flap procedures leave scars both where the tissue was taken and on the reconstructed breast.

Reconstruction won't make a "perfect" breast. The goal is to make the size and shape of your breasts look alike so you'll feel comfortable when you wear clothes. You will be able to see the difference between your reconstructed breast and your other breast when you are naked.

You will have less feeling in your reconstructed breast. Nerves and feelings in the nipple and skin of your breast are affected by breast surgery.

Questions to ask the doctor about breast reconstruction

1. Could I have breast reconstruction?

2. What types of reconstruction could I have?

3. What is the average cost of each type? Does insurance cover them?

4. What type of reconstruction is best for me? Why?

5. How should I expect the reconstructed breast to look?

6. Will I have any feeling in my reconstructed breast?

7. What possible side effects should I know about?

8. How much pain will I feel?

9. How long will I be in the hospital?

10. Will I need blood transfusions for the procedure? If so, can I donate my own blood?

More questions on next page

11. How long will it take me to recover?

12. When would I be able to do things like driving and working?

13. What kinds of changes to my breast can I expect over time?

14. What happens to my breast as I get older, or if I gain or lose weight?

15. Are there any new reconstruction options that I should know about?

Is my cancer gone forever?

What if my cancer comes back?

Sometimes breast cancer does come back. You need to know that this doesn't happen to many women.

In some women, a few cancer cells live through treatment and grow into tumors. The cancer can recur (come back) where it first started or in your other breast. It also can come back in the lungs, liver, brain, lymph nodes closest to the breast, and bones. Some things to remember:

- **It's normal to worry about the chance that your cancer may come back.**

- **Don't wait to talk to your doctor** about anything happening in your body that worries you.

- **Everyone has aches and pains.** Most of the time they aren't a sign that cancer is back. If the pain gets worse and lasts for a few weeks, call your doctor.

- **You'll probably feel better with each visit to your doctor.** Be sure to see your doctor. Get regular checkups after treatment. They may help you get on with your life without worrying too much about whether the cancer will come back.

Can I lower my chances that the cancer will come back?

Some medicines may lower your chance of breast cancer coming back.[15]

Because these drugs have side effects, you and your doctor will need to discuss them. Here are some medicines to discuss with your doctor:

- **Tamoxifen** (sold under the brand names **Nolvadex, Istubal,** and **Valodex**) has been used for several years to lower the risk that breast cancer will come back. Many studies show that taking tamoxifen for five years lowers a woman's chance of cancer coming back. Your doctor can tell you about side effects.

- **Anastrozole (Arimidex), letrozole (Femara), and exemestane (Aromasin)** are newer, hormone-type medicines that may be used instead of tamoxifen to stop cancer from coming back in women who have gone through menopause. These drugs also cause side effects.

- **Chemotherapy** drugs like **paclitaxel (Taxol)** or **docetaxel (Taxotere)** are also being tested to find out if they can lower the chance that cancer will come back when they are used with other drugs after surgery.

How will I know if my cancer comes back?

See your doctor for regular checkups. This is the best way to check for any signs your cancer has come back.

If cancer does come back, it usually happens within a few years of a woman first finding out she has breast cancer. That's why it's so important after treatment to see your doctor on a regular schedule. Follow these steps:

- **After treatment,** look for any changes in your body. Tell your doctor about anything new or strange.

- **Have a mammogram every year.** Having a mammogram is really important for women after breast cancer treatment. If you have had a lumpectomy, radiation, or chemotherapy, you may need a mammogram every six months for a while. If you have had certain kinds of mastectomy, you may not need to have mammograms on that side of your body anymore. Ask your doctor.

- **Have a doctor check your breasts each year.** Mammograms don't reveal every tumor. Get checked each year. And pay attention to your own breasts. Tell your doctor about any lumps, bumps, or other changes you find.

When should I call the doctor?

Call the doctor about any changes you find or pain you have. Also, call if you have any questions.

Talk with your doctor about the following issues:

- Changes in your body you think may be a sign that cancer has come back

- Any pain you have

- Any problems that bother you or stop you from living your normal life. These include fatigue, trouble sleeping, not wanting to have sex, or gaining or losing weight.

- Any medicines, vitamins, or herbs you are taking, and any other treatments you are using

- Any strong feelings you have, like being worried or depressed

- Any changes in the health of your family, especially if someone else gets cancer

Questions to ask the doctor about checkups and cancer coming back

1. How often should I see you for checkups?

2. How will you check me for cancer?

3. What changes in my body should I watch for?

4. Will insurance cover my checkups?

5. Am I at high risk for my cancer coming back?

6. Is there anything I can do to lower the chances of my cancer coming back?

7. Could medicine help lower my chances of cancer coming back?

125

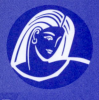

How can I be close with someone after cancer and treatment?

Recovering

How will cancer and treatment affect my sex life?

It may take time for you to want to have sex again.

Many women find that they don't want to have sex during treatment. They may be thinking too much about other things. Some treatments may make you less interested in sex. See how you feel. Just know that it's okay to have sex during and after treatment.

You and your partner may need time to get used to being together again. Take the time you both need to feel relaxed. There are different ways to be close, like holding each other. After treatment, your partner may be afraid to have sex after everything you've gone through. You may need to be the one to say when you want to hug, kiss, and make love.

Talk about what you are afraid of or what bothers you. If you admit that you feel worried about being close or having sex, your partner may be able to give you the support you need. It may help if both of you try these suggestions:

- Relax
- Have fun
- Be honest about how you feel
- Talk about what the other person could do to make you feel better
- Keep a sense of humor

Should I talk about my cancer with someone new I'm dating?

Wait until you're comfortable with the person. Then be honest.

You may not want to talk about your cancer. Or you may worry that someone you're dating won't want to be with you because you've had cancer. Keep in mind the following:

- Telling a date within a few minutes of meeting is probably too soon. But if you wait until you are about to get into bed to tell a partner that you've had surgery on your breast, you risk shocking the person.

- Wait until you are both relaxed and feeling close to talk about your cancer.

- Share that you have had cancer if you get serious with someone, especially if cancer has affected how long you may live or whether you can have children.

Even people without cancer may reject each other because of looks, beliefs, personalities, or other reasons. Sadly, some dates may reject you because of your cancer. You could avoid being rejected if you stayed at home and didn't date. But you'd also miss the chance to be happy with another person. A loving partner will love both you and your history.

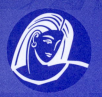

How can I stay healthy from now on?

What can I do to keep my body healthy?

You can eat right and exercise, drink less, and not smoke.

You couldn't control your cancer, but you can do things to make your health better after cancer:

- Eat right
- Exercise
- Drink less alcohol, if you drink at all
- Quit smoking

Taking the steps above is a good idea for anyone who wants to live a healthy life. We cannot say for sure that taking these steps will keep your cancer from coming back, but they may help. And they can help keep you from getting another type of cancer.

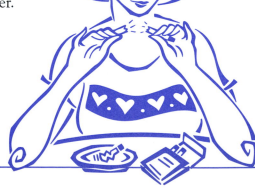

How can I eat right after cancer treatment?

Eat lots of healthy foods, such as fruits, vegetables, and whole grains.

Having a healthy weight is more important than ever. Eating healthy will help you keep a healthy weight if you are currently overweight.

- Choose foods and beverages in amounts that help you maintain a healthy weight.
- Eat five or more servings of vegetables and fruits each day.
- Choose whole grains instead of processed (refined) grains and sugars.
- Limit the amount of processed and red meats that you eat.

Eating a diet made up of mostly vegetables, fruits, and whole grains is good for your health and can help reduce cancer risk. And eating five or more servings of vegetables and fruits each day is easy when you consider how small one serving really is:

- $^1/_2$ cup cooked vegetables
- 1 cup leafy vegetables
- $^3/_4$ cup 100% juice
- 1 medium-size piece of fruit
- $^1/_2$ cup fruit
- $^1/_4$ cup dried fruit

See also page 155 to find out how much food makes up one serving.

Low-fat and fat-free don't always mean low-calorie. Low-fat foods that are high in calories from sugar and other substances will not help control your weight. Try eating vegetables, fruits, and whole grains instead of higher-calorie foods.

Eating right and being active go hand in hand. Watching what and how much you eat and being more active are keys to weight control. Try to balance the amounts of calories you eat with exercise.

Call the American Cancer Society at **800-ACS-2345 (800-227-2345)** for more information on eating healthy and staying active.

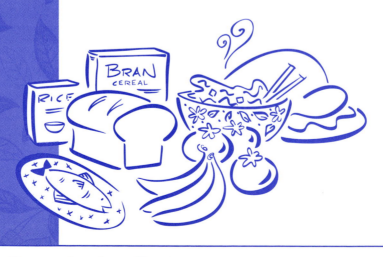

How should I exercise after cancer treatment?

Talk to your doctor first. Find out what kinds of exercise are safe for you. Then have fun exercising.

Exercise can help you feel like you're in charge of your body again. It also can help you feel good about reaching your activity goals. Exercise helps you build stronger muscles, become more flexible, and have more energy. You may feel more relaxed and positive after exercising. Follow these exercise tips:

- **Talk to your doctor before you start exercising.** Find out what kinds of exercise are safe and healthy for you.

- **Don't overdo it.** Start slowly for just a few minutes a day if you haven't exercised in a while or if you haven't exercised before. You will get stronger.

- **Try to be active for forty-five minutes, five times a week.** Have fun and pick exercises you like. Choosing exercise that you like will help you stick with it and reach your activity goals.

- **Stretch before you exercise,** do your exercise, slow down before you stop to cool down, and stretch after you stop.

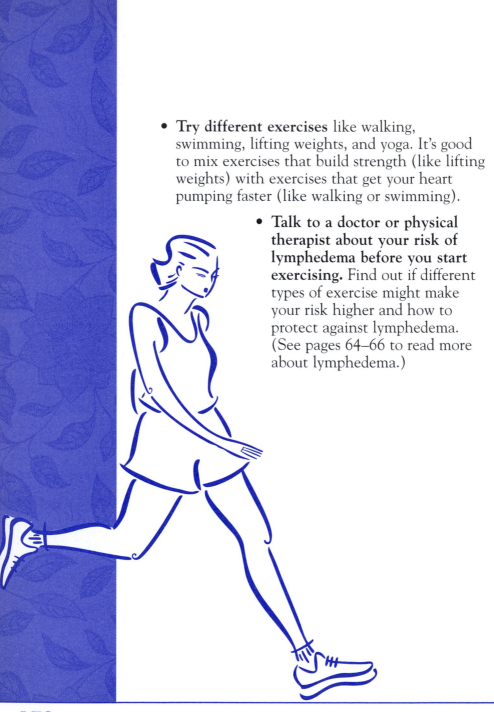

- **Try different exercises** like walking, swimming, lifting weights, and yoga. It's good to mix exercises that build strength (like lifting weights) with exercises that get your heart pumping faster (like walking or swimming).

  - **Talk to a doctor or physical therapist about your risk of lymphedema before you start exercising.** Find out if different types of exercise might make your risk higher and how to protect against lymphedema. (See pages 64–66 to read more about lymphedema.)

How can I get back to living my life?

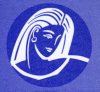

Can I live a normal life again?

You can live a full and happy life after treatment.

You are a woman who had cancer, but there is more to your life than that. Doing the things that have always made you happy may make you feel better and more normal now. If you feel like it, go out and enjoy yourself.

After dealing with breast cancer and treatment, you may feel tired. You may have forgotten what it was like to take care of yourself. Try some of the ideas below to feel normal again and make yourself happy.

Express yourself:

- **Laugh.** Watch a funny movie or spend time with a friend who makes you smile.

- **Share your thoughts and feelings** by painting, writing in a journal, singing, or dancing.

- **Talk to someone you trust.** Find someone you feel safe with—a partner, friend, sister, religious leader, or counselor—and really let out your thoughts and feelings.

Do things for you:

- **Work your mind.** Read a book, take a class, or try a new hobby.

- **Take time alone.** Set a time each day or week to do just what you want to do.

- **Do nice things for yourself.** Check out books from the library, rent a movie, ask your partner to give you a foot massage, or take a hot bath.

Think about what's important:

- **Decide what really matters** and let go of the "small stuff."

- **Tap into your faith.** Join a prayer group at your place of worship if you belong to one. Find prayers you like and say them often.

- **Set limits.** Think about your work duties, your chores around the house, and your social life. Then set some limits. Cut back on activities until you are doing only what matters most and what brings you the most rewards.

What do I do now?

You decide what happens in your life now.

Sometimes having cancer makes people think about their lives in a different way. You may not worry so much about little problems. You may want to spend more time with the people you love and less time at work or doing housework. Or you may realize how important your family, job, free time, or friendships are to you.

Think about coming up with a list of simple things you can do to make your life better. Be specific. Here are some ideas:

- Eat a family dinner together three nights a week with no TV.
- Call a loved one once a week.
- Volunteer with a cancer support group one day a month.
- Learn to dance, paint, or play an instrument.
- Read a book you've always wanted to read.
- Plan a vacation to a beautiful place.
- Go visit an old friend.
- Spend an hour by yourself once a week and do whatever you want.

Cancer may have shown you that each day you are alive is a gift. It is up to you to make each day what you want it to be.

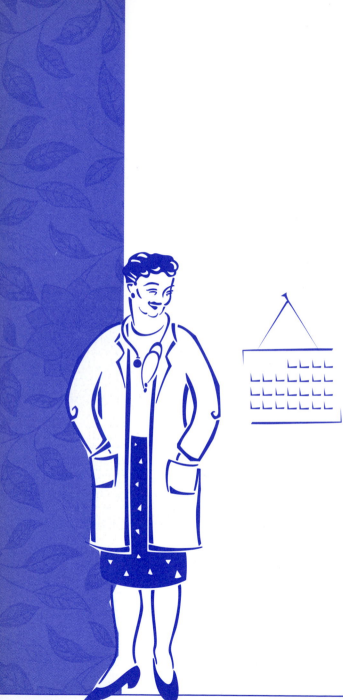

More Information

How should women get checked for breast cancer?

If you have had breast cancer, your doctor will tell you how often you should go in for checkups after treatment.[16]

If you are worried about the health of your women family members and friends, show them the list below. It explains how they should get checked for breast cancer. Although most women don't get breast cancer, a woman's chance of getting breast cancer increases as she gets older. Also, if you have a mother, daughter, or sister, her chances of getting breast cancer are greater now that you have had breast cancer. She should talk to her doctor about how often she should get checked for breast cancer. Talk to her about the first item below.

1. **Women who have a higher risk of breast cancer** should talk with their doctors. Their doctors may want them to start having mammograms (x-rays of the breast) before they are forty years old. Their doctors also may want them to have other tests or get checked for breast cancer more often than other women.

2. **Women who are in their twenties and thirties** should have their breasts checked by a nurse or doctor once every three years. This can be done during a regular checkup at the doctor's office.

3. **Women who are forty years old and older** should have their breasts checked by a nurse or doctor once every year. This can be done during a regular checkup.

4. **Women who are forty years old and older** should also schedule a mammogram once every year.

5. **Women of any age** should tell their doctors about any changes they notice in their breasts right away. Women in their twenties should start checking their own breasts for any changes. Nurses and doctors can teach women how to check their breasts for lumps or changes. If your doctor doesn't talk to you about a breast self-exam, ask how to do it.

Can you help me understand breast cancer risk?

What does it mean if I am "at risk" for breast cancer?

Being "at risk" for breast cancer has to do with things that increase your chances of getting breast cancer.[17]

A risk factor is something in your life that increases your chance of something happening, like getting breast cancer. Any woman could get breast cancer, but the things listed on the next page can increase a woman's chances of getting the disease.

The idea of risk factors can be confusing. Just because a woman has one or more risk factors for breast cancer doesn't mean that she will get breast cancer. Even if risk factors increase the chances that breast cancer could grow, they don't mean that breast cancer will grow.

Some women who have a risk factor (or many risk factors) never get breast cancer. In fact, most women who do get breast cancer don't have any risk factors.

What risk factors increase a woman's chances of getting breast cancer?

There are two kinds of risk factors that can increase a woman's chances of getting breast cancer.

The first type of risk factors are ones that women cannot change in their lives. Here are some examples:

- Being a woman
- Getting older, especially over fifty years of age
- Having a sister, mother, or daughter who has had breast cancer

The second type of risk factors are related to lifestyle. Here are some examples:

- Not having children
- Having a first child after thirty years of age
- Using birth control pills
- Not breastfeeding
- Drinking two or more drinks of alcohol a day
- Taking hormone replacement therapy (also called HRT)

Are other women in my family more likely to get breast cancer?

Your mother, sisters, or daughters do have a higher chance of getting breast cancer.

Some breast cancers "run in families." This means that if one woman in your family has breast cancer, the other women in your family have a higher chance of getting it too. If, in addition to you, your mother, sister, or daughter also has breast cancer, the risk is even higher for your other female relatives. Here are other factors that increase your risk:

- If anyone in your family had breast cancer at the age of forty-nine or younger
- If anyone in your family had ovarian cancer

If this describes your family, tell your close female relatives to talk with their doctors. Doctors may want them to start having mammograms and other tests when they are young.

Remember, the fact that you have breast cancer doesn't mean that other members of your family will get breast cancer. It means that their risk is higher than that for women without breast cancer in their families.

See pages 137–138 to find out how healthy women should get tested for breast cancer.

Can anything lower a person's chances of getting breast cancer?

Yes. Some things may lower the risk of getting breast cancer.

If you have breast cancer, you may want to know how to help your friends and loved ones lower their risk of getting breast cancer. These tips may also help lower your risk of having breast cancer come back.

Here are some guidelines:

- Keep a healthy weight instead of being overweight
- Exercise each day
- Drink less alcohol
- Eat lots of fruits and vegetables and less red meat

Living a healthy life can help a woman lower her chances of getting breast cancer. It doesn't mean she won't get breast cancer, but it might help. And taking the steps above also helps lower her chances of getting heart disease and diabetes.

I've heard that smoking and breast implants can increase your chances of getting breast cancer. Is that true?

Many of the beliefs people have about what causes breast cancer are not true[18]:

- **The world around us:** Most experts believe that air and water pollution has very little effect on breast cancer risk.

- **Abortion or miscarriage:** Having an abortion or a miscarriage has not been shown to increase the risk of breast cancer.

- **Smoking:** Studies don't prove that smoking leads to a higher risk for getting breast cancer. But not smoking improves your overall health and lowers the risk of getting other cancers, heart disease, and stroke.

- **Antiperspirants:** Using underarm antiperspirants or regular deodorants has not been shown to increase risk. These products are tested to make sure they are safe.

- **Getting hurt:** A breast injury does not increase cancer risk.

- **Underwire bras:** Bras with underwires do not increase breast cancer risk.

- **Breast implants:** Breast implants do not increase breast cancer risk.

How can I have breast cancer if no one in my family has had it?

Women who don't have a family member with breast cancer can still get breast cancer.

Women who do not have a close relative with breast cancer may still get breast cancer. You may be the first person in your family to get breast cancer. Most breast cancer occurs in women who do not have any other close family member with it.

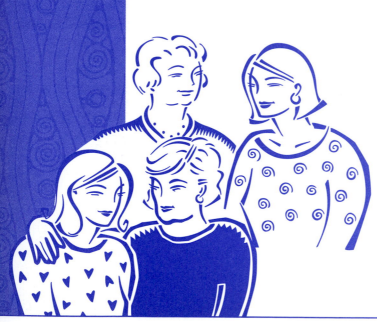

More about cancer grades

"Cancer grade" means how likely it is that your cancer will grow and spread quickly. Your cancer will be given a grade from 1 to 3.

Grade 1 cancer cells look the most like normal cells and are the least likely to grow and spread quickly. Grade 3 cancer cells look the most different from normal cells. They are more serious and could grow quickly.

More about cancer stages

On my pathology report, what do the letters T, N, and M and the numbers 0, 1, 2, 3, and 4 mean?

These letters and numbers tell you how much and where the cancer has spread in your body.

The letters T, N, and M are used to describe the size of your tumor and how much it has spread.

- **T** stands for the size of the cancer.

- **N** stands for any cancer that has spread to the lymph nodes near the breast. Lymph nodes are small bean-shaped areas of tissue that help fight infections in the body.

- **M** stands for cancer that has spread to other areas of the body.

Numbers follow each of these letters. Lower numbers mean you have a smaller tumor or a tumor that has not spread much or at all. Higher numbers mean you have a larger tumor or a tumor that has spread more.

- **T0, T1, T2, T3, and T4:** T0 is the smallest and least serious tumor, while T4 is the biggest and most serious.

- **N0, N1, N2, and N3:** N0 shows the least spread to the lymph nodes and is the least serious. N3 has spread widely to the lymph nodes and is the most serious.

- **M0 and M1:** M0 means the cancer has not spread to other areas of the body, and M1 means cancer has spread to other areas.

My doctor says I have stage IIIA breast cancer. How are the letters T, N, and M and the numbers 0 to 4 related to the stage?

They are related. Doctors use the T, N, and M categories to figure out one number and letter that describes your cancer stage, such as IIIA.

Doctors will look at each of the T, N, and M categories of your cancer before deciding on the overall stage of your cancer.

When doctors figure out your overall cancer stage, they don't talk about the T, N, and M categories anymore. They use a shortcut: a single Roman numeral and a letter.

Every woman's breast cancer is said to be one of these stages: stage 0, stage I, stage IIA, stage IIB, stage IIIA, stage IIIB, stage IIIC, or stage IV.

Stages are shown as:

- 0 (the least serious), I, II, III, or IV (the most serious) and

- A (the least serious), B, or C (the most serious)

- Ask your doctor what your cancer stage means for your health, your treatment options, and your future.

What's the difference between my stage IIB breast cancer and my friend's stage IIIC breast cancer?

Breast cancer is more serious if it is described by a higher stage number and letter.

Someone whose cancer has grown and spread a lot will have higher numbers in each of the T, N, and M categories. Her cancer also will be a higher overall stage. This means she has a more serious cancer than someone whose cancer has not grown and spread as much (and who has a lower overall stage). Here are some examples:

- Someone whose cancer is T2, N1, and M0 has stage IIB breast cancer.

- Someone whose cancer is T4, N2, M0 has stage IIIC breast cancer. She has a more serious cancer than a woman with stage IIB breast cancer. Her T number, which means her tumor size, and N number, which has to do with if the cancer has spread to lymph nodes, are more serious than the T and N numbers of the woman with less serious stage IIB breast cancer.

Your medical team

You will have many health professionals and support staff working with you during your breast cancer diagnosis, treatment, and recovery. Here's a list describing members of your cancer care team:

Anesthesiologist *(an-es-thee-zee-OL-uh-jist)*

An anesthesiologist is a medical doctor who gives anesthesia (drugs or gases) to put you to sleep. These drugs also help prevent or relieve pain during and after surgery.

Medical Oncologist

A medical oncologist is an expert in cancer care and treatment. This doctor will help you make decisions about your treatment. He or she may keep in contact with other members of your medical team to make certain you are receiving the best treatment possible. Your oncologist will follow up with you during your treatments.

Nurses

Several different nurses may care for patients with breast cancer. A **registered nurse** can monitor your condition, provide treatment, tell you about side effects, and help you adjust to the effects of breast cancer. A **nurse practitioner** shares many tasks with your doctors, such as recording your medical history, conducting physical exams, doing follow-up care, and even writing prescriptions (with the doctor's supervision). A **clinical nurse specialist (CNS)** may provide special services, such as leading support groups. An **oncology nurse** has a great deal of knowledge about cancer care and may work in several areas.

Pathologist *(path-OL-uh-jist)*

A pathologist is a medical doctor who has been trained to diagnose disease by looking at tissue and fluid samples. He or she will determine the classification (cell type), help determine the stage (extent) of your cancer, and write a pathology report so that you and your doctor can decide on treatment options.

Personal or Primary Care Physician

A personal physician may be a general doctor or have special training in gynecology, internal medicine, or family practice. He or she is often the medical doctor who examined you when and if you had symptoms of breast cancer. This doctor will talk with you about your breast cancer and will be involved in your care. Your personal or primary care physician provides details of your medical history to other members of the team. He or she also will refer you to breast cancer care specialists.

Physical Therapist/Physiotherapist
(*fiz-e-o-THAYR-uh-pist*)

A physical therapist is a trained health specialist who helps you regain strength and movement after surgery. The physical therapist teaches you exercises and other ways to strengthen your body. He or she may use massage or heat to help you restore or maintain your body's strength, function, and flexibility.

Plastic Surgeon/Reconstructive Surgeon

A plastic surgeon/reconstructive surgeon is a medical doctor who performs operations to restore parts of the body affected by injury, disease, or treatments for cancer. You may consult with him or her before and after breast cancer surgery. Your plastic/reconstructive surgeon can perform breast reconstruction during or after a mastectomy.

Radiation Oncologist

A radiation oncologist is a medical doctor who treats cancer with radiation (high-energy x-rays). He or she will decide what kind and how much radiation you should receive after your lumpectomy or mastectomy, or to control advanced breast cancer. This member of your medical team checks on you often during and after treatment.

Radiation Therapist

A radiation therapist is a trained technician who works with the radiation oncologist (see page 152). He or she positions your body during the treatment and gives you the radiation therapy.

Radiologist

A radiologist is a medical doctor who has special training in the use of x-rays, mammography, ultrasound, and other imaging procedures. He or she has special training in diagnosing breast cancer and other diseases. Your radiologist writes a radiology report to your personal doctor, medical oncologist, radiation oncologist, or surgeon describing the findings. The radiology images and report may be used to aid in diagnosis, to help locate tumors during surgery and radiation treatment, or to help classify and determine the extent of your breast cancer.

Radiology Technologist

A radiology technologist is a trained health professional who assists the radiologist. He or she is trained to position you for x-rays and mammograms and to develop and check the images for quality. The images taken by your radiology technologist are sent to your radiologist to be read.

Social Worker

A social worker will help you and your family deal with emotional and practical problems, such as finances, child care, emotional issues, family concerns and relationships, transportation, and problems with the health care system. Your social worker may have special training in cancer-related problems and can provide counseling, answer questions about treatment, and lead cancer support groups.

Surgeon

A surgeon is a medical doctor who performs surgery. You will consult with your surgeon before and after you undergo a lumpectomy, biopsy, or other surgical procedure. The surgeon will remove tumors and, if necessary, surrounding tissue. Your surgeon works closely with other members of your medical team. He or she will give a surgical report to your personal doctor and to your radiation and medical oncologists that will help determine your future treatment plan.

What counts as a serving?

Part of eating healthy is knowing how much food you're eating. Use this chart to find out what makes a serving of different foods. Each of the following items counts as one serving:

Fruits

- 1 medium apple, banana, or orange
- $1/2$ cup of chopped, cooked, or canned fruit
- $3/4$ cup of 100% fruit juice

Vegetables

- 1 cup of raw, leafy vegetables
- $1/2$ cup of other cooked or raw vegetables, chopped
- $3/4$ cup of 100% vegetable juice

Grains (choose whole grains when you can)

- 1 slice of bread
- 1 ounce of ready-to-eat cereal
- $1/2$ cup of cooked cereal, rice, or pasta

Beans and nuts

- $1/2$ cup of cooked dry beans
- 2 tablespoons of peanut butter
- $1/3$ cup of nuts

Dairy foods and eggs

- 1 cup of skim or low-fat milk or yogurt
- $1 1/2$ ounces of natural low-fat cheese
- 2 ounces of processed low-fat cheese
- 1 egg

Meats

- 2 to 3 ounces of cooked lean meat, poultry, or fish

Resources that may help

These are groups around the country that can give you information or support. You also may find breast cancer information and support services in your area. Ask your doctor or check your phone book or the Internet for nearby sources of help.

You can get in touch with most of these groups by phone, fax, or e-mail, and sometimes through Web sites. Keep in mind that new Web sites appear every day while old ones change, move, or disappear. Some of the Web sites below, or what they offer, may be different by the time you read this book. A simple Internet search will often show you the new Web site for a group.

About the Internet

There is endless information about cancer and related topics on the Internet. This can be helpful when you are choosing what to do about your health. But think about where the information comes from. Is the group that provides the information respected? Can you trust what they say? Are they trying to sell you anything? Always talk about health information you find on the Internet with your doctor. He or she can help you figure out if this is information you can trust.

Cancer Information and Services

American Cancer Society

250 Williams Street NW • Atlanta, GA 30303-1002
Toll-free: 800-ACS-2345 (800-227-2345)
Call anytime day or night; English and Spanish available
Web site: http://www.cancer.org

The American Cancer Society is a voluntary health organization that works all over the United States. It counts on volunteers in local areas to help. The Society works to prevent cancer, find cancer early, save lives, and ensure that fewer people suffer from cancer. They work toward this goal through research, teaching people, supporting the government's role, and helping people affected by cancer. The Society gives people information about cancer, has programs for patients, and helps people find help in their area.

National Cancer Institute

NCI Public Inquiries Office • 6116 Executive Boulevard
Room 3036A • Bethesda, MD 20892-8322

Toll-free: 800-4-CANCER (800-422-6237)
Web site: http://www.cancer.gov

This government agency provides consumers and patients with
cancer information. The NCI has many publications about
cancer. Some publications are offered in Spanish. You also can
call the toll-free number (800-422-6237) for information about
where to get a mammogram in your area.

The Susan G. Komen Breast Cancer Foundation

5005 LBJ Freeway, Suite 250 • Dallas, TX 75244

Toll-free (helpline): 800-I'M-AWARE (800-462-9273)
Phone: 972-855-1600 • Fax: 972-855-1605
Web site: http://www.komen.org

The Susan G. Komen Breast Cancer Foundation is an
international nonprofit organization dedicated to eradicating
breast cancer as a life-threatening disease by advancing cancer
research, education, screening, and treatment. Their Web site
offers news and information on breast health, drug treatments,
treatment options, educational events and meetings, survivor
stories, and other breast cancer-related information.

Help with Paying Medical Bills and Other Costs

U.S. Social Security Administration

Office of Public Inquiries • Windsor Park Building
6401 Security Boulevard • Baltimore, MD 21235

Toll-free: 800-772-1213
Web site: http://www.ssa.gov

The Social Security Administration runs the Supplemental
Security Income (SSI) program. They can tell you how to
apply for Social Security Disability Income (SSDI).

Help with Getting Treatment, Mammograms, and Medications

American Association of Retired People (AARP)
601 E Street NW • Washington, DC 20049

> Toll-free: 888-OUR-AARP (888-687-2277)
> Web site: http://www.aarp.org
> Web site (for help with medications):
> http://www.aarppharmacy.com/aarpNet

This organization offers membership to anyone over fifty years old. They charge a small yearly fee. AARP focuses on the needs of older people across the U.S. Their Web site includes information on a service that offers discounts on drugs.

Eldercare Locator
The Administration on Aging
U.S. Department of Health & Human Services

> Toll-free: 800-677-1116
> Web site: http://www.eldercare.gov

Eldercare Locator is a service available all over the U.S. It helps senior citizens and those who care for them find local support and help with transportation, meals, housing, home care, and legal issues.

ENCORE Plus Program of the YWCA Office of Women's Health Initiatives

> Toll-free: 800-953-7587
> Phone: 202-467-0801
> Web site: http://www.ywca.org

This breast and cervical cancer program provides information and mammograms to women who are in need and don't have access to breast health services. Free services include teaching about breast and cervical cancer and help finding low-cost or free exams to check for breast cancer. Search for "breast cancer screening" at the Web site above or call the toll-free number to find a program in your area.

Hill-Burton Program

U.S. Department of Health and Human Services
Health Resources and Services Administration

Toll-free: 800-638-0742
Toll-free in Maryland: 800-492-0359
Web site: http://www.hrsa.gov/hillburton/default.htm

Depending on the size of your family and how much money you make, you may be able to get help paying for your health care through the Hill-Burton program. You can apply for Hill-Burton at any time, before or after you have care. Call the number above to find a Hill-Burton facility near you. Then ask to speak to someone in the admissions, business, or patient accounts office there. They can tell you how to apply for Hill-Burton.

Medicare Hotline

U.S. Department of Health & Human Services

Toll-free: 800-MEDICAR (800-633-4227)
Web site: http://www.medicare.gov

This hotline offers information about who can be part of Medicare, how to sign up, what is covered, payment and billing, insurance, prescription drugs, and frequently asked questions. Call to get information about services in your area.

National Breast and Cervical Cancer Early Detection Program (NBCCEDP)

Centers for Disease Control and Prevention (CDC)

Toll-free: 888-232-6348
Web site: http://apps.nccd.cdc.gov/cancercontacts/
nbccedp/contacts.asp

NBCCEDP helps women in need get free or low-cost mammograms as well as get checked for cervical cancer. There are programs in every state and U.S. Territory. Call the number above or go to the Web site to find out where you can get a mammogram.

NeedyMeds

P.O. Box 63716 • Philadelphia, PA 19147

Phone: 215-625-9609 • Fax: 419-858-7221
Web site: http://www.needymeds.com/newuser.html

NeedyMeds can give you information about where to get help paying for medicines. They will help you find out if you may be able to get the medicines you need for free through a patient assistance program.

The Partnership for Prescription Assistance

Toll-free: 888-4PPA-NOW (888-477-2669)
Web site: http://www.pparx.org

Patient assistance programs offer free or lower cost medicines to people whose prescription drugs aren't paid for by insurance. This program offers people access to more than 275 assistance programs. Call or go to the Web site to find out which programs you could be part of. You can call for forms or get forms online to apply. The American Cancer Society is a national partner in this program. Information is available in Spanish.

Pharmaceutical Research and Manufacturers Association of America (PhRMA)

950 F Street NW • Washington, DC 20004

Phone: 202-835-3400
Fax: 202-835-3414
Web site: http://www.phrma.org

PhRMA provides information about pharmaceutical companies that are part of PhRMA and drugs that are currently available, being tested, or being developed. The Web site includes a list of patient assistance programs for prescription drugs.

U.S. Department of Veterans Affairs Benefits Office

Toll-free: 800-827-1000
Web site: http://www.va.gov

If you are a veteran of the armed forces or married to a veteran, you may be able to get health care through the Department of Veterans Affairs. The number above connects you to your local office.

U.S. Social Security Administration
Office of Public Inquiries
Windsor Park Building
6401 Security Boulevard • Baltimore, MD 21235

Toll-free: 800-772-1213
Web site: http://www.ssa.gov

Call the toll-free number to learn about services in your area, SSI, or SSDI. Or visit the Web site to learn more about benefits, disability, and other information.

Traveling to Treatment and Places to Stay

If you have Medicaid you can get help with travel plans or costs for getting to and from medical centers and doctors' offices for treatment. You may be paid back for gas, get help paying for bus fare, or you may be able to use a vanpool. Talk to your Medicaid eligibility worker about options.

Community and church groups may also be able to help with travel or paying for it. Talk to a social worker at the hospital about other help. You may even be able to get help with paying for parking at the hospital.

Many treatment centers have places you can stay for a little while or can help with lower costs at nearby motels and hotels. Ask the social worker or nurse where you're getting treated for ideas on low-cost housing during treatment.

American Cancer Society Hope Lodges
American Cancer Society

Toll-free: 800-ACS-2345 (800-227-2345)
Web site: http://www.cancer.org (search for "Hope Lodge")

The Hope Lodge offers short-term housing for people who are in cancer treatment and their family members. Hope Lodges offer comfortable rooms, kitchens, and may offer help with getting to and from treatment.

Road to Recovery and Other Transportation Programs
American Cancer Society

Toll-free: 800-ACS-2345 (800-227-2345)

In this American Cancer Society program, available in some areas, volunteers drive patients and family to hospitals and clinics for treatment. In some parts of the country, the program may also offer help paying for gas. Call to find out what is available in your area.

Westin Hotel Guestroom for Cancer Patients

Toll-free: 800-ACS-2345 (800-227-2345)

Along with the American Cancer Society, some Westin hotels will provide rooms when cancer patients must travel to receive treatment. Some rooms are free. Others are offered at lowered rates.

Wigs, Prostheses, and Makeup

Look Good…Feel Better
American Cancer Society
Cosmetic, Toiletry and Fragrance Association Foundation (CTFA)
National Cosmetology Association (NCA)

Toll-free: 800-395-LOOK (800-395-5665)
Web site: http://www.lookgoodfeelbetter.org

This free program can teach you how to look and feel beautiful during chemotherapy and radiation treatment. Certified beauty professionals offer tips on makeup, skin care, nail care, and head coverings.

tlc (Tender Loving Care)
American Cancer Society

Toll-free: 800-850-9445 • Fax: 800-279-2018
Web site: http://www.tlcdirect.org

This American Cancer Society catalog offers special products and information for women with breast cancer who are dealing with losing hair and other side effects of treatment. The catalog offers affordable mail-order products like wigs, hats, and prostheses.

Support for You and Your Loved Ones

CancerCare

275 7th Avenue, Floor 22 • New York, NY 10001

Toll-free (Counseling): 800-813-HOPE (800-813-4673)
Phone: 212-712-8400 • Fax: 212-712-8495
E-mail: info@cancercare.org
Web site: http://www.cancercare.org
Site in Spanish: http://www.cancercare.org/espanol

This nonprofit group offers free programs for counseling, information, and practical help. CancerCare can help people with cancer, their families, and friends cope with cancer and its effects. Spanish-speaking staff is available.

Cancer Survivors Network (CSN)

American Cancer Society

Toll-free: 877-333-4673 (877-333-HOPE)
Web site: http://www.acscsn.org

If you can get on the Internet, you can get in touch with other women with breast cancer, their families, and friends through this American Cancer Society program. CSN was created by and for cancer patients and their families. CSN is made up of people who have been affected by cancer and would like to share strength and hope. It is private and safe. You can listen to other people's stories, make your own Web page, or "chat" with other people.

I Can Cope

American Cancer Society

Toll-free: 800-ACS-2345

I Can Cope is an American Cancer Society program for people with cancer and the people who take care of them. The program offers information, support from others, and tips on how to cope.

Reach to Recovery
American Cancer Society

Toll-free: 800-ACS-2345

Reach to Recovery is an American Cancer Society volunteer program. Women who have had breast cancer give support to women with breast cancer and their loved ones. Survivors can talk to you in person or over the phone. They are trained to help when you are being diagnosed or during treatment, if your cancer comes back, and when you are getting better after treatment. Visits are always free.

Self-Help for Women with Breast or Ovarian Cancer (SHARE)
1501 Broadway, Suite 704A • New York, NY 10036

Toll-free: 866-891-2392
Breast hotline: 212-382-2111
Latina hotline: 212-719-4454
Fax: 212-869-3431
Web site: http://www.sharecancersupport.org

SHARE operates three hotlines for anyone who is worried or has questions about breast or ovarian cancer. Hotline volunteers are breast or ovarian cancer survivors. SHARE offers information about breast cancer and emotional support. It also can help you find groups all over the U.S. Spanish-speaking staff is available.

Y-Me National Breast Cancer Organization
212 West Van Buren, Suite 1000 • Chicago, IL 60607

Toll-free hotline: 800-221-2141
Toll-free Spanish hotline: 800-986-9505
Phone: 312-986-8338 • Fax: 312-294-8597
Web site: http://www.y-me.org
Web site (Spanish version): http://www.y-me.org/espanol

Y-Me teaches and supports people with breast cancer and their families. Y-Me provides a 24-hour hotline, groups that can help, support groups for men and women with breast cancer, a newsletter, a library, information on treatment centers and hospitals, and help finding wigs and prostheses. Spanish-speaking staff is available.

Young Survival Coalition (YSC)

61 Broadway, Suite 2235 • New York, NY 10006

Toll-free: 877-YSC-1011
Phone: 646-257-3000
Fax: 646-257-3030
E-mail: info@youngsurvival.org
Web site: http://www.youngsurvival.org

The YSC is a nonprofit group of breast cancer survivors and supporters all over the world. The YSC aims to help women forty and under who have breast cancer. It is also a way for young women who are living with breast cancer to find each other.

How You Can Help Others

Tell A Friend

American Cancer Society

Toll-free: 800-ACS-2345 (800-227-2345)

Through Tell A Friend, you can volunteer to support your friends and family by reminding them to get a mammogram. Call to learn more about breast cancer or about being a Tell A Friend volunteer.

Glossary

alternative treatments: anything that is said to treat or cure cancer when in fact it has not been proven to be a treatment for cancer. They can be powerful and may hurt you. They haven't been strictly tested by scientists or have been tested and have been shown not to work.

antiperspirants (*an-TEE-per-spe-rants*): deodorants that stop you from sweating.

areola (*uh-REE-uh-luh*): the dark area around the nipple.

benign (*buh-NINE*): not cancer. Tumors can be either cancer or benign. Not all lumps or tumors are cancer; some are benign.

biopsy (*BY-op-see*): taking out some tissue, such as from the lump in your breast. Doctors look at the sample of tissue and cells under a microscope to find out if a person has cancer and to learn more about it.

breast cancer: cancer that starts in the breast. Cancer cells in the breast are growing and forming new cells without stopping or dying like healthy cells do.

breast conservation therapy: treatment aimed at saving or conserving the breast; it involves having a lumpectomy and radiation therapy.

breast form: also called a prosthesis. It is padding shaped like a breast or part of a breast that can be worn in your bra to fill it out after breast surgery.

breast implant: a padding filled with saline (salt water) or silicone gel that is put just under the skin where breast tissue was removed. This padding fills out the shape of your breast.

breast reconstruction: surgery that can rebuild the shape of a woman's breast, including her nipple and areola.

breast self-exam: how women check their own breasts for changes that could be cancer. Doctors and nurses can teach women how to do this.

cancer: cells that keep changing and growing out of control. Healthy cells in your body grow, form new cells, do what they are supposed to do in your body, and later die. But cancer cells keep growing, forming more cells, and spreading in the body. They don't die like other cells.

cancer grade: how likely it is that your cancer will grow and spread quickly. Breast cancer is given a grade of 1 to 3, with 1 the least serious and 3 the most serious.

cancer stage: how much cancer is present in the body and if it has spread. Doctors use a code of letters and numbers to describe how much cancer has spread.

cell: all living things, from plants to people, are made up of tiny cells.

chemotherapy *(kee-moh-THAYR-uh-pee)*: drugs that kill cancer cells. They are either put into the body with needles or swallowed as pills. They stop cancer cells from growing and dividing wherever they are in the body.

diagnosis *(die-ug-NO-sis)*: when the doctor finds out you have cancer.

fatigue *(fuh-TEEG)*: a very tired feeling that can be caused by cancer treatment. It is different than being tired from not having enough sleep. It is feeling like your brain, body, and emotions are all tired. This is the most common side effect of cancer treatment.

flap procedure: breast reconstruction in which a doctor uses tissue from somewhere else in your body to make what looks like a breast. The tissue can come from your tummy, back, hip, or buttocks.

hormones: chemical substances released into the body by the endocrine glands. Hormones travel in the blood and set in motion certain body functions. Testosterone and estrogen are examples of male and female hormones. Certain kinds of breast cancer need hormones so they can grow.

hormone replacement therapy (HRT): taking hormones after you have gone through menopause, when your body stops making hormones.

hormone therapy: cancer treatment with hormones or with drugs that interfere with hormone production or action. This is not the same as hormone replacement therapy (HRT). Hormone therapy also may involve surgery to take out hormone-producing glands. Hormone therapy may kill cancer cells or slow their growth.

insurance benefit: the medical care, drugs, and supplies covered by health insurance.

insurance claim: the bills you or your doctor send to the insurance company so they will pay them.

lumpectomy (*lump-EK-tuh-me*)**:** taking out a cancerous lump and some of the breast around it, but not the full breast.

lymphedema (*limf-uh-DEE-muh*)**:** a buildup of lymph fluid that causes the arm to swell.

lymph (*limf*) **nodes:** small bean-shaped areas of tissue that help fight infections in the body. Cancer can spread in the body through lymph nodes. Doctors may remove some lymph nodes to find out if there is cancer in them.

malignant (*muh-LIG-nunt*)**:** cancer.

mammogram: an x-ray picture of the inside of your breast.

mastectomy (*mas-TEK-tuh-me*)**:** removing all of the breast or both breasts (double mastectomy).

menopause: when a woman stops having her period and her body stops making hormones.

metastasis (*meh-TAS-tuh-sis*)**:** when cancer cells break away and spread to other, distant parts of the body.

monoclonal antibody (*ma-nuh-KLO-nul ANN-tih-bah-dee*)**:** like proteins but made in a lab and put into the body. They stop cancer cells from growing by stopping proteins from working right. They don't hurt healthy cells.

nauseated (*NAW-ze-at-ed*)**:** feeling sick, like you might throw up.

nipple reconstruction: a type of breast reconstruction where tissue for the nipple and areola is (1) taken from a patient's body, usually from her upper inner thigh, and shaped into a nipple, or (2) where small flaps of skin on the reconstructed breast are brought together to form the nipple. Tattooing may be used to match the nipple of the other breast and create the areola.

oncologist (*on-CALL-uh-jist*)**:** a doctor who treats people with cancer.

pathology (*path-AWL-uh-gee*) **report:** a report that explains the type of breast cancer you have, how big the tumor is, and if it's likely to grow quickly. Doctors write the report based on what they see when looking at the tissue under the microscope. They use the report as a guide to help plan how to treat your cancer.

patient assistance programs: programs that offer free or lower cost medicines to people whose prescription drugs aren't paid for by insurance.

prognosis (*prog-NO-sis*)**:** how doctors think your cancer will probably grow and what your chances are of recovering.

prosthesis (*pross-THEE-sis*)**:** also called a breast form. It is padding shaped like a breast or part of a breast that can be worn in your bra to fill it out after breast surgery.

proteins: proteins made by your body help it grow, fix itself when it's hurt, stay healthy, and do other important things.

radiation (*ray-dee-AY-shon*) **therapy:** treatment with special x-rays that kill or shrink cancer cells. A special machine is used to point x-rays at the cancer to kill or hurt cancer cells. Sometimes it can be given by putting tiny pellets into the body where the cancer is, or by using a needle to put radioactive material into the body where the cancer is.

recurrence: cancer that comes back after treatment.

remission: when tests don't show any cancer after treatment. Cancer seems to be gone.

risk factor: something in your life that changes your chances of something happening, like getting breast cancer.

side effects: unwanted things that happen because of treatment, like losing hair because of chemotherapy or feeling tired from radiation therapy.

supplement: a vitamin or mineral that doesn't come from foods but comes in pills, for example.

tissue: cells that work together to do a certain job in the body.

tumor (*TOO-mer*)**:** cells that form a lump in the body. Tumors are sometimes cancer and sometimes not.

x-rays: low levels of radiation that make a picture of the inside of the body. X-rays are used in mammograms. High levels of x-rays can be used in radiation therapy to kill cancer cells.

Endnotes

1. American Cancer Society. Overview: Breast Cancer. What Causes Breast Cancer? Revised 09/26/2006. http://www.cancer.org/docroot/ CRI/content/ CRI_2_2_2X_What_causes_breast_cancer_5.asp?sitearea= Accessed March 5, 2007.

2. American Cancer Society. *A Breast Cancer Journey*, *2nd ed*. 2004, p. 49.

3. American Cancer Society. *A Breast Cancer Journey*, *2nd ed*. 2004, p. 75.

4. American Cancer Society. *A Breast Cancer Journey*, *2nd ed*. 2004, p. 67.

5. American Cancer Society. *A Breast Cancer Journey*, *2nd ed*. 2004, p. 74.

6. American Cancer Society. Overview: Breast Cancer. How Is Breast Cancer Treated? Revised September 9, 2006. Available at: http://www.cancer.org/docroot/CRI/content/CRI_2_2_4X_How_Is_Breast_Cancer_Treated_5.asp?sitearea=. Accessed March 5, 2007.

7. American Cancer Society. Overview: Breast Cancer. How Is BreastCancer Treated? Revised September 9, 2006. Available at: http://www.cancer.org/docroot/CRI/content/CRI_2_2_4X_How_Is_Breast_Cancer_Treated_5.asp?sitearea=. Accessed March 5, 2007. BreastCancer.org. Lumpectomy: Breast-conserving surgery. Available at: http://www.breastcancer.org/ tre_surg_conssurg.html Accessed February 26, 2007.

8. American Cancer Society. *A Breast Cancer Journey, 2nd Ed*. 2004, pp. 241-243.

9. American Cancer Society, National Endowment for Financial Education. In Treatment. Financial Guidance for Cancer Survivors and Their Families. No. 35001-Rev August, 2006. Available at: http://www.cancer.org/downloads /CRI/In_Treatment.pdf. Accessed March 5, 2007.

10. Medical Insurance and Financial Assistance for the Cancer Patient. Revised April 9, 2006. Available at: http://www.cancer.org/docroot/MLT/content/MLT_1x_Medical_Insurance_and_Financial_Assistance_for_the_Cancer_Patient.asp. Accessed March 5, 2007.

11. American Cancer Society. A *Breast Cancer Journey*, 2nd ed. 2004, pp. 179-189.

12. American Cancer Society, National Endowment for Financial Education. In Treatment. Financial Guidance for Cancer Survivors and Their Families. No. 35001-Rev August, 2006. Available at: http://www.cancer.org/downloads/ CRI/In_Treatment.pdf. Accessed March 5, 2007.

13. American Cancer Society. A *Breast Cancer Journey*, 2nd ed. 2004, pp. 203-225.

14. American Cancer Society. Detailed Guide: Breast Cancer. What Happens After Treatment for Breast Cancer? Revised September 18, 2006. Available at: http://www.cancer.org/docroot/CRI/content/CRI_2_4_5X_What_happens_after_treatment_5.asp?sitearea=. Accessed March 5, 2007.

15. American Cancer Society. A *Breast Cancer Journey*, 2nd ed. 2004, pp. 165-178.

16. American Cancer Society. Breast Cancer: Early Detection. American Cancer Society Recommendations for Early Breast Cancer Detection in Women Without Breast Symptoms. Revised September 21, 2006. http://www.cancer.org/docroot/CRI/content/CRI_2_6x_Breast_Cancer_Early_Detection.asp?sitearea=. Accessed March 5,2007.

17. American Cancer Society. Overview: Breast Cancer. Can Breast Cancer Be Prevented? Revised September 26, 2006. http://www.cancer.org/docroot/CRI/content/CRI_2_2_2X_Can_breast_cancer_be_prevented_5.asp?sitearea=. Accessed March 5, 2007.

18. American Cancer Society. A *Breast Cancer Journey*, 2nd ed. 2004, pp. 25-26.

Books published by the American Cancer Society

Available everywhere books are sold and online at
www.cancer.org/bookstore

Inspirational Survivor Stories

Angels & Monsters: A child's eye view of cancer

*Crossing Divides: A Couple's Story of Cancer, Hope,
and Hiking Montana's Continental Divide*

I Can Survive (Illustrated)

Praise for *Angels & Monsters:*

"Stunningly beautiful and thought-provoking… Sensitive,
insightful, unique and thoroughly "kid-friendly." Highly
recommended reading for any child [and parent] having to
cope with cancer, and would make a welcome and valued
addition to any school or community library collection."
—*Midwest Book Review*

Praise for *Crossing Divides:*

"Every life has its mountains to climb. Read on and find the
inspiration to reach your summit."
—*Bernie Siegel, MD*

"The challenges of confronting the dangers and frustrations
of the wilderness become a metaphor in this fascinating
book for facing the challenges of a cancer illness. …Love of
life and love of nature are fused into a remarkable human
experience that ensures the reader will find new meaning in
juxtaposition with illness."
—*Jimmie C. Holland, MD, Chair,
Department of Psychiatry & Behavioral Sciences,
Memorial Sloan-Kettering Cancer Center*

Support for Families and Caregivers

Cancer in the Family: Helping Children Cope with a Parent's Illness

Caregiving: A Step-by-Step Resource for Caring for the Person with Cancer at Home, Revised Edition

Couples Confronting Cancer: Keeping Your Relationship Strong

When the Focus Is on Care: Palliative Care and Cancer

Praise for *Caregiving:*

"A thorough and accessible resource."

—*Former First Lady Rosalynn Carter, Author,* Helping Yourself Help Others

"Chock-full of sensible and reassuring information, easily accessible to the average reader. Good glossary and extensive resource section included. Recommended."

—*Library Journal*

"...Designed for caregivers but is equally informative for the patient. Well-organized."

—*Bookpage*

Help for Children

Because...Someone I Love Has Cancer:
    Kids' Activity Book

Mom and the Polka-Dot Boo-Boo

Our Dad Is Getting Better

Our Mom Has Cancer
    (available in hard cover and paperback)

Our Mom Is Getting Better

Praise for *Our Mom Has Cancer*:

"I needed a way to let my children know what they could expect as far as my therapy, and let them know what might happen emotionally. ...Excellent, and I would recommend it to any parent who has been diagnosed..."

—*A mom from Cedar Rapids, Iowa*

Tools for the Health Conscious

ACS's Healthy Eating Cookbook, Third Edition

Celebrate! Healthy Entertaining for Any Occasion

Good for You! Reducing Your Risk of Developing Cancer

The Great American Eat-Right Cookbook

Kicking Butts: Quit Smoking and Take Charge of
    Your Health

National Health Education Standards: Achieving
    Excellence, Second Edition

Health Books for Children

Healthy Me: A Read-Along Coloring & Activity Book

Kids' First Cookbook: Delicious-Nutritious Treats to Make Yourself!

Praise for *Kids' First Cookbook:*

"A cookbook with a contemporary look filled with nutrition information. The uncluttered…layout is pleasing and employs colored type, drawings, and helpful photographs. A solid effort that will encourage healthy eating habits."

—*School Library Journal*

Information for People with Cancer

Site-Specific

ACS's Complete Guide to Colorectal Cancer

ACS's Complete Guide to Prostate Cancer

A Breast Cancer Journey, Second Edition

QuickFACTS™ Colon Cancer

QuickFACTS™ Lung Cancer

QuickFACTS™ Prostate Cancer

Symptom Management

ACS's Guide to Pain Control, Revised Edition

Eating Well, Staying Well During and After Cancer

Lymphedema: Understanding and Managing Lymphedema After Cancer Treatment

Praise for *QuickFACTS™ Lung Cancer:*

"The ACS has achieved its goal of providing overviews that tackle need-to-know issues and supply references for additional follow-up information as desired. Recommended."

—*Library Journal*

Praise for *Lymphedema:*

"Written in a supportive and accessible voice, the book [Lymphedema] will be most useful to those who have been touched by lymphedema and who are seeking comprehensive and authoritative coverage of their concerns. Recommended for public and consumer health libraries."

—*Library Journal*

Cancer Information

The Cancer Atlas
    (available in English, Spanish, French, Chinese)

Cancer: What Causes It, What Doesn't

Coming to Terms with Cancer: A Glossary of Cancer-Related Terms

Informed Decisions, Second Edition

The Tobacco Atlas, Second Edition
    (available in English, Spanish, French, Chinese)